LOVERS

&

SURVIVORS

A Partner's Guide to

Living With and Loving

a Sexual Abuse Survivor

D1598458

by

S. Yvette de Beixedon, Ph.D.

Robert D. Reed Publishers • San Francisco, California

Robert D. Reed Publishers

750 La Playa, Suite 647 • San Francisco, CA 94121

Telephone: (415) 997-4567 • Fax: (415) 997-3800

Book Cover by Destiny Design

Editing, Typesetting, and Layout by Pamela D. Jacobs, M.A.

Library of Congress Cataloging-in-Publication Data
de Beixedon, S. Yvette.
    Lovers & survivors : a partner's guide to living with and loving a sexual abuse survivor / by S. Yvette de Beixedon.
    p.   cm.
    Includes bibliographical references.
    ISBN 1-885003-09-9 : $14.95
    1. Adult child sexual abuse victims--Mental health. 2. Adult child sexual abuse victims--Family relationships. 3. Inter-personal relations. 4. Intimacy (Psychology) I. Title. II. Title: Lovers and survivors.
RC569.5.A28B45   1995
616.85'82239--dc20   94-43251
                                          CIP

Manufactured, Typeset, and Printed in the United States of America

Dedication

In loving memory
of Pauli

without whom this book
could not have been published.

Note of Thanks

I am grateful to all of the clinicians whose research facilitated the development of this book, and I would like to extend my special appreciation to Christine A. Courtois, Ph.D., Wendy Maltz, and Beverly Holman, for their permission to incorporate selections of their work into this guide.

Acknowledgments

There is no way that I can pay tribute to all of the people who supported me in the development and publication of this book. But, I would like to honor a few of these very special folks:

to the men and women who must remain nameless—who generously allowed me to tell their courageous stories, so that others could engage in the healing process.

to Evette Ludman—who was there at the very inception of these ideas and encouraged me to put them on paper.

to Jane Amsler—who kept me going when I thought that dawn would never come.

to Mary McNaughton Cassill—who painstakingly read through the manuscript and gave me her thoughtful input.

to Jeffrey Schlicht—who offered technical and emotional support during the publication process.

to Jennifer White—with whom I have laughed and cried, and shared some of my deepest and darkest hours, and who watched me come into my own during the process.

to John—who was there in the beginning, making me laugh, in spite of myself.

to my parents—who have shared their adult lives with me, and have learned to support me in the most emotionally generous ways.

to my Nana and Grandpa—to whom I owe my life. Their wisdom, serenity, kindness, and stability has nourished my growth and enabled me to emerge triumphant.

and to my husband—whose shining inner flame renewed my cooling embers. Richard, thank you for your patience, guidance and boundless emotional support. Your belief in me and this book means the world. I look forward to forever with you.

Contents

Informational Highlights

Exercises

Preface

Why write a book for partners only?

Partners are the unsung heroes in the survivor's life, often sitting behind the scenes—nurturing, caretaking, even thinking for the survivor at times. A partner is the rock that a survivor may choose to cling to. A partner is the one she or he pushes away, then holds on to tightly. A partner may be the only one to see the tears, the anger, or the craziness. And a partner may be the one to witness the joy, the pride, and the ecstasy of healing.

Research on sexual abuse has been conducted only within the last few decades. Currently, there are numerous resources for survivors to use in their efforts for healing. However, research and writing for and about partners has only taken off within the last few years.

The partner's time has come. It's the partner's turn to learn, develop, grow, and blossom. Now you, as a partner, can have a chance to learn about yourself—about how you interact with your partner, what to expect of your relationship, and how your partner's survival affects you as an individual and as a partner.

This book offers information, encouragement, and resources to the partner who wants to participate in the healing process. Sexual abuse can impact anyone at any time; therefore, the book provides examples for both male and female survivors.

Who is the author?
What does she bring to this book?

Dr. S. Yvette de Beixedon is a licensed psychologist who specializes in the treatment of sexual abuse survivors and their partners. She has practiced in all regions of the United States and has worked with survivors and their partners from all walks of life.

Introduction

What you are getting into

Healing from child sexual abuse spans a lifetime. While professional intervention (especially early help) can promote healing, the scars of this injury never disappear. Your partner will continue to heal and recover throughout his/her life—sometimes moving forward in a linear fashion and, at other times, sliding backwards. Healing requires the courage of self, friends, and family. The courage to heal is sometimes hard to come by. If you have culled some courage in order to confront your own abuse, or the abuse of your partner, you are wise. And if these confrontations generate further courage, you can share your inner power with someone else who has yet to find that courage.

Living and loving with a survivor is not for the faint of heart. It takes work, and unceasing willingness to continue growth and development of the relationship for its lifetime. Flexibility and compassion must become household words, as the survivor learns to integrate his/her traumas and joys into an "accepted self." Empathy and understanding are prerequisites for harvesting love and warmth between you and your partner.

As a couple, you must work together to develop a healthy relationship which can support both of you as individuals; and one which can provide a warm, safe place when the rest of the world is in an uproar. Your partner is trying to heal; and, therefore, you will probably have to nurture and comfort your partner, as well as offer strength, sustenance, and fun—even when you may feel exhausted and depleted. The survivor, too, must make an effort to reach out to you, to accept what you have to offer, and to learn to give back to you, as she or he mends her or his wounded soul.

While you may not have been abused yourself, by uniting with your partner, you have become a "survivor- by-association" or a "co-survivor." While you may not experience the same challenges and obstacles presented to your partner, you will struggle with your own dilemmas, feelings, and thoughts. The two of you must take steps together to heal and grow. Those steps may be unfamiliar and uncomfortable at times, but if both of you are willing to try and willing to compromise, the process can be managed. Never forget: you are in this together.

This book is divided into three main sections. In Section One, you will read about "Getting to know your partner." When you feel more knowledgeable about sexual abuse and its effects on your partner, you can begin to consider the factors in Section Two—those factors required for "Developing a healthy relationship with your partner." Finally, when you have a better idea of what you *do* know, you will begin to recognize the areas in which you need help. Section Three is about "Asking for help and using it to your benefit."

Reading this material may be difficult at times, so I encourage you to get support to make it through the entire book. Stop and take a break whenever you need to, even if it is for a week or a month. If you decide that you cannot continue your relationship after weighing all of the factors, then read this material for yourself.

Survivors are everywhere. It is unlikely that your partner is the only survivor with whom you will ever have contact. Allow yourself to know about sexual abuse. Give yourself permission to learn more about yourself and your partner. Read to gain wisdom, strength, and healing.

"I Believe You"

Out of the night
>There comes a voice,
>>She says,
>>>"Believe me."

And, so
>I believe her
>>With all of my love,
>>>And all of my strength
>>>>And all of my voice.

For her
>And for all the years
>>That the voice was
>>>Mine
>>And no one
>>>Believed me.

For all of those I believe in,

S. Yvette de Beixedon, Ph.D.

Post script:

I do this job because I love it. I do this work because I must. I must believe in them, because this belief is a necessity of our common survival.

Section I

Getting To Know Your Partner

You have developed an intimate relationship with your partner, and you have discovered that she or he is a survivor of sexual abuse. What do you do now?

As in all relationships, it is important that you really get to know your partner. So far, you may feel as if you have some idea of who your partner is. Perhaps you know her or his favorite color, book, movie, or food. Perhaps you share favorite activities with your partner or you know just where to take her or him after a hard day at work. Maybe you are still discovering and exploring little details. Even if you have discussed some aspects of who your partner is, how much do you really know? Have you seen a glimpse of the Big Picture yet? Most partners have a difficult time getting to know their partner, so I have written a book to help with this process.

Get to know your partner. Ask her or him to describe her or his life, ideas, feelings, and thoughts. At the same time, begin reading and learning some of the basics about sexual abuse and healing. As you read, you may find that you recognize your partner in the following pages.

Chapter 1
Sexual Abuse 101:
Basic Information About Sexual Abuse

- What is sexual abuse? How is it defined?
- What percentage of the population is sexually abused? What percentage is impacted by it?
- How and why does sexual abuse affect children and adolescents differently (and often more severely) than it does adults?
- Where, when, and how does it happen?
- Who does it? To whom? Why?
- What is the prognosis?

Definitions and Statistics

As the universal silence of sexual abuse is slowly broken with each new day, definitions become broader-based and more applicable to all. While I hope to define sexual abuse in a fresh way that will generate insight for each person who reads this book, the inherent concept of sexual abuse has remained the same through time. At the very least, I can provide you with some of the most recent definitions and statistics for sexual abuse.

Things have changed remarkably in the last century. From an era in which sexual abuse was almost unheard of (it existed, it just wasn't discussed!), we have entered an era in which survivors are encouraged to speak out and toddlers are taught from a very early age to protect their physical boundaries from disrespectful strangers by saying, "No!" or "Stay away from me!" Even children in day care and nursery school are taught the difference between "good touch" and "bad touch." Preschools now teach their students to develop a password with their parents and guardians so that the children can distinguish dangerous strangers from representatives sent by the parent (e.g. to pick up the child from school). Yet, even in this era, sexual abuse is perpetuated. For every two children who learn to say, "Get away from me!" to that adult stranger there is another child who learns the message, "This is our secret. Don't tell!"

Statistics

Within the last five years recognition of sexual abuse and its effects on survivors has mushroomed. After decades of silence, survivors are finding a safe and supportive environment in which to reveal their long-kept secrets in order to heal their wounded, traumatized "inner children," causing statistics for sexual abuse to rise exponentially.

In 1984, it was estimated that as many as 50% of the adult female population and as many as 10% of the adult male population report chronic sexual abuse as children. When people are taught how to identify sexual abuse, an even greater number report histories of abuse. Today, accepted estimates suggest that one in every two women and one in every four men has been or will be sexually abused during his/her lifetime.

In addition, sexual abuse and abuse recovery do not occur in a vacuum. If we consider all of the partners, family members and friends who experience victimization or survival "by association," the percentage of the population which is affected by sexual abuse is overwhelming. If you're reading this book, you've probably already experienced the grave proximity of sexual abuse in your life. For those readers who are still unsure whether or not they are survivors themselves or are interacting with a survivor, a definition of sexual abuse might be helpful.

Definition

The term "sexual abuse" incorporates physically, verbally and psychologically abusive behaviors. For instance, while many people may believe that sexual abuse is limited to sexual touching or intercourse with preteen children, it actually spans a much broader spectrum.

The older brother who taunts his young sister about the unattractive physical proportions of her body as he watches her disrobe, both demeans and demoralizes her while violating her right to privacy. The mother who maintains her toddler's hygiene by inserting soap into his anus during his daily bath violates her son's physical boundaries and rationalizes it as health care. The baby sitter who rubs his clothed or exposed genitals on his young charge's body or face is introducing the child or adolescent to behaviors and emotions for which the child is not yet prepared to manage, generating unnecessary and potentially harmful confusion and distress.

All of these actions may be perceived as sexually abusive; and unfortunately, examples come from all walks of life. Children of both genders, and of all socioeconomic levels, races, religions, ethnic backgrounds, cultures, and nationalities are abused. Child sexual abuse touches individuals from infancy to late adolescence. Perpetrators include but are not limited to:

- parents
- siblings
- relatives
- friends
- neighbors
- baby-sitters
- day care workers
- teachers
- coaches
- medical practitioners
- religious mentors
- employers
- mail carriers
- Scout leaders
- household staff

Types of Sexual Abuse

Examples for sexual abuse can include contact and non-contact behaviors that range from verbal and psychological harassment to rape. Verbal abuse may be generated by a variety of individuals. One daughter recalled the abuse spouted by her mother:

> *"I see how you look at your father. You want to fuck him! Well, go ahead, you two belong together! Why don't you just fuck him right here, you slut!"*

Another client recalled the psychological abuse she endured from her father:

> *"You're never going to please any man with those little tits! You're not even good enough to look at! You make me want to retch. Why don't you see if you're brother wants you? He might be able to show you some tricks so you can get a guy some day!"*

Contact sexual abuse may range from incidental touching (i.e. during bathing) and observation (such as watching a child or adolescent disrobe for the observer's own gain) to vaginal or anal rape. The range of sexual abuse includes but is not limited to:

- willfully appearing nude in front of a child or an adolescent
- disrobing in front of the child or adolescent
- forcing the child or adolescent to disrobe
- exposing one's genitals to the child or adolescent
- watching the child or adolescent (i.e. while bathing)
- kissing the child or adolescent for sexual pleasure
- fondling or touching the child or adolescent
- masturbating in front of the child or adolescent
- performing oral sex on the child or adolescent
- forcing the child or adolescent to perform oral sex
- forcing the child or adolescent to engage in "dry intercourse" (e.g. rubbing one's genitalia on the child or adolescent without penetration)
- penetrating the anus or vagina of the child or adolescent with a finger or object
- penetrating the anus or vagina of the child or adolescent with the penis

This continuum of sexual behaviors ranges from non-contact actions to distinct sexual contact. This ranking of behaviors does not suggest that those at the beginning of the list are any less abusive than those near the end of the list. While there are some common responses to many forms of sexual abuse, the impacts of abuse really depend on the survivor and his/her experiences.

Child Victims

"Sexual contact does not have to be violent, painful, or always unwanted to constitute abuse. It is abuse if victims are robbed of their sexual innocence and manipulated into premature sex for someone else's benefit." [1] Abusers may manipulate their victims by threatening them directly, or they may use subtler coercion if they already have a relationship with the child which is characterized by a large power differential (e.g. authority figure and child). The child may be "further coerced by the perpetrator's strong desire to keep the activity a secret, which has the purpose of minimizing intervention and allowing repetition." [2]

Manipulation of power or status is only one of the methods by which children and adolescents become vulnerable to abuse. Additionally, while some abusers believe that their child victims consented to sexual activity, most societies have laws which assert that children are never capable of giving sexual consent to an adult. If the perpetrator convinces the child of his/her consent to sexual acts, the child's sense of guilt and/or shame may then be used as "leverage" by the perpetrator to maintain the abuse. A perpetrator may also manipulate a child by offering or withdrawing privileges, acceptance, and love to maintain the cooperation of the child.

Guilty feelings are especially common for the child who willingly participates in the abuse in order to attain affection or attention when these are otherwise unavailable. In an age in which children often live in single-parent families or in families in which both parents work outside the home, children are often left feeling empty and disconnected. Kelsey struggles with her need for affection:

> *I know what you're saying is right. I know he abused me. But I went to him! I can't get over that he hurt me and I went back for more! It's just that I had nothing else. Mom was always at work. There was no one else to love me. There wasn't even anyone to notice me. I took anything I could get— no matter how much it hurt me.*

While the abuser may interpret the child's willingness as consent, it can not be considered free consent in any sense. "When a power imbalance exists because of differences in age and sexual sophistication, real consent cannot exist." [3]

Another reason children respond differently than adults to sexual abuse is that they lack a comprehensive language to describe the abuse to others. While "most survivors knew something was wrong with the contact, [they] lacked the maturity needed to identify what was wrong and to express it." [4]

While some children are unable to accurately explain what has happened to them due to their limited linguistic skills, other children are abused prior to the development of any language and may never be able to verbalize their pain and shame. These survivors often experience the same deficits and strengths common to many survivors, but may never gain access to visual memories of the abuse. Survivors who endured abuse pre-verbally are capable of feeling the impacts of the abuse and may even develop thoughts and beliefs similar to survivors who were abused after developing language.

Survivors who were abused prior to middle adolescence do not generally have a sense of themselves or their identity in the world. They may understand little of what is actually happening to them or what their options might be. They rarely have the ability to understand the complexities of adult sexuality and consenting interaction. For these reasons, children are often unable to recognize the dangerous situations in which they may become entrapped and they are most likely unaware of "escape routes" available to them in those situations.

We move now to the definition and statistics currently available on incest—the form of sexual abuse which is most likely to be chronic and to remain "hidden" from all those outside of the incestuous relationship.

Incest

It has been said that, "Incest lacks all the essential conditions for positive, healthy sexuality. There is not true consent, equality, respect, trust, or safety. Incest perpetrators use their victim's age, dependence, and immaturity to their advantage. Because incest is universally regarded as wrong and harmful, practically all cultures have laws that forbid it. Incest is considered a deviant type of sexual behavior that warrants labeling the perpetrator a social criminal in need of behavioral restraint." [5]

Statistics

Recent research suggests that incest is the most common form of sexual abuse. It has been suggested that at least 20% of all women endure at least one incestuous experience prior to the age of eighteen, and that nearly 5% of the female survivors were abused by their fathers. Of those women, it is likely that half of them will not remember the incestuous experience until memories are sparked, or "popped," in adulthood.

In her book, *Healing the Incest Wound*, Dr. Courtois notes that females, who constitute the majority of abuse survivors, are more likely to be abused by a family member, while males are more likely to be abused by someone outside the family.

Incest rarely involves the use of physical violence. Russell, whose research is summarized in Dr. Courtois' first book, found that only 32% of the sample reported that they had endured physical violence during the abuse. Of this group, 29% indicated that they had been pushed or pinned down, 2% reported being hit or slapped, and 1% were beaten. More commonly, perpetrators use verbal threats to coerce the child to submit to and/or to maintain the incest.

Defining Incest

The "typical" pattern of incest is described as repeated sexual contact which is initiated prior to puberty and lasts for several years. The contact generally become progressively more intrusive, often culminating in some form of penetration by the perpetrator. While current research suggests that most children are abused between the ages of seven and twelve, the age of onset of abuse is probably quite a bit younger. Children who are sexually abused during early childhood do not have the cognitive, emotional or psychological resources to manage the experience of sexual abuse and more than likely repress, deny or forget their experiences in order to cope.

Additionally, incest survivors may minimize their distress in order to hide their shame (of participating in activities that they experienced as "wrong" or "bad") and/or to protect the family member who abused them (for more information about how children protect their perpetrators, read about the process of "trauma bonding" described in the works of Jan Hindman). We are generally hopeful that children who are raised in this new era of awareness will report incest sooner, putting an end to the abuse, and providing us with clearer descriptions and parameters for incest.

The most comprehensive definition for incest (with a female victim) currently available is provided below:

> [Incest] refers to sexual contact with a person who would be considered an ineligible partner because of his blood and/or social ties (i.e. kin) to the subject and her family. The term encompasses, then, several categories of partners, including father, stepfather, grandfather, uncles, siblings, cousins, in-laws, and what we call "quasi-family."

The last category includes parental and family friends (e.g. mother's sexual partner). Our feeling is that the incest taboo applies in a weakened form to all those categories in that the "partner" represents someone from whom the female child should rightfully expect warmth or protection and sexual distance" (here partner refers to the sexual partner rather than the survivor's current spouse or mate).[6]

Other researchers have added that perpetrators described above are generally, but not always, five to forty years older than the children that they abuse. While abuse by a perpetrator who is older or physically larger than the child may be easy to identify, it may be more difficult for a parent, relative, teacher or support provider to identify and empathize with peer incest. Peer incest refers to sexual contact between individuals who are closely matched by age and genetics (e.g. older siblings, cousins, step- and half-siblings), which is non-mutual and/or forced.

While many may believe that sexual "exploration" between peers is "harmless," if the contact is non-consenting (at what point does the child even know to what he/she is consenting anyway?), the trauma incurred by age mates can be just as serious as that generated by older perpetrators.

In addition to peer incest, individuals may be abused by those in their nuclear (parents or siblings) and extended families (grandparents, uncles, aunts, cousins). Children may be abused by both same-sex and opposite-sex perpetrators, and may even be sexually abused by more than one member of the family ("multiple incest"). For more information about these categories of abuse, read *Healing The Incest Wound* by Christine Courtois.

All of the behaviors which were previously described (in the beginning of this chapter) as sexually abusive also apply to incestuous abuse. In fact, four of the five examples offered earlier reflected abuse by a relative.

Some investigators also believe that the effects of incest far outweigh the effects of non-incestuous abuse due to the destruction of a significant, protective relationship between the child and his/her abuser. Others have added that, while children may prepare themselves in some minute way for the danger associated with strangers, children rarely learn to guard themselves against the violations of relatives. As a result, it has been suggested that these kind of sexual transgressions shock and traumatize the child to a greater extent than those personal violations about which the child has been educated and sensitized.

How Does Incest Happen?

Family Influences and Dynamics

Incestuous families often seem OK. When teachers and friends discover incest in a family, they often comment on how normal and "together" the family appeared. When these incested families are more closely examined, a veritable web of furtive, convoluted relationships is revealed. In their book, *Incest and Sexuality*, Wendy Maltz and Beverly Holman describe families who harbor incest as a team of "rock climbers connected by ropes that scale the side of a mountain, all family members are integrally connected in a journey through time."

While the strategically covert actions of incested families resemble those of rock climbing squads in their efforts to effect survival of the unit, they differ in one primary function. Climbing squads work synergistically for the benefit of each individual's survival. Families harboring incest survive parasitically, maintaining the unit at the expense of specific members of the family (covertly, and often unconsciously, selected to be the scapegoat-victims).

Many investigators believe that child sexual abuse occurs in a step-wise progression, rather than as an impulsive single episode. Generally, the perpetrator first identifies or locates his child victim. Often the abuser is a person with whom the child has occasional or frequent contact, thus providing both access and opportunity for the perpetrator. I am reminded of a recent case in the news which described a Scout leader's use of Scout meetings to gain access to children whom he would later approach and sexually abuse. The relationship of the Scout to his Scout master accurately reflects the adult's abuse of power: the Scout perceives his leader in a position of authority, and submits to the leader's requests/demands because he trusts his leader to uphold the Boy Scout Promise, "to do my duty to God and my Country and obey the Scout Law to help other people at all times, to keep myself physically fit, mentally awake, and *morally straight.*"

In addition to the abuse of power, the abuser may induce children subtly or more forcefully. Many abusers become quite adept at identifying the "soft spots" of their prey and may, for example, readily provide attention to the neglected child in exchange for sexual favors from the child, as did Kelsey's perpetrator. Additionally, perpetrators often disguise the sexual activity as a "game," and children may not understand what is happening to them at the time. If the perpetrator's position of authority, or affectionate exchanges are insufficient to gain the compliance or submission of the child, the abuser may revert to more forceful coercion or violence.

The Process of Incest

Once the perpetrator has access to a child, the sexual abuse begins. At first the perpetrator may limit abuse to non-contact behaviors such as having the child watch the perpetrator stimulate him/herself, or asking the child to pose for nude photographs. The abuse generally becomes more intrusive and may progress from oral penetration to vaginal or anal penetration. Each instance of child sexual abuse is individualized, and has its own rules and parameters. Therefore, if you or your partner did not experience such a progression, it doesn't mean that it wasn't abuse, it just means that the abuse was a little different from the norm.

After the onset of the abuse, the perpetrator must gain the child's silence, through threat, intimidation, or emotional disadvantage. Because of the taboos against talking about sexual abuse, children who may want to speak out, do not. Members of incested families maintain the silence together in order to avoid facing the horrifying reality existing in their home.

The Child's or Adolescent's Response

In the incested family, the child occupies an inferior, even submissive, and powerless position. When that child is abused, he/she experiences even more overwhelming helplessness (in response to the failure of the perpetrator to heed the child's requests for the abuse to stop). Helplessness then transforms into self-blame and guilt as the perpetrator convinces the child of his/her consent to the sexual acts. This sense of guilt and/or shame may then be used to perpetuate the abuse. The child who is "taught" then, that he/she is responsible for the abuse, experiences his/her own *entrapment*, and must then learn to *accommodate* to the potentially chronic sexual abuse, and will most likely not disclose the abuse to others, due to her feelings of self-blame. Some of the ways in which children learn to cope and accommodate are described in Chapter 2.

Maintenance of Chronic Abuse

The perpetrator will attempt to maintain the abuse in any way he/she can. To the abuser, the sexual abuse is very satisfying: he/she gains sexual pleasure and fulfillment, a sense of power and dominance, mastery of a relationship which requires few of the demands of an adult relationship, and may increase the perpetrator's self-esteem. In order to maintain his/her satisfaction, the perpetrator must coerce the child to stay silent about their activities. Sometimes, the attention and affiliation that the neglected or isolated child experiences are sufficient to maintain the sexual abuse. In other cases, the perpetrator may threaten the child with anger, blame, separation (e.g. "If you tell, I'll have to go away and won't be able to play with you anymore"); abandonment ("If you tell, your parents won't love you anymore and they'll give you away!"); sexual abuse of others (e.g. "If I can't have you, I guess I'll have to start up with your sister/brother"); or harm to self and/or significant others (e.g. "If you tell, I'll kill myself!" or "If you tell anyone, I'll kill your parents/siblings/pets!"). Sometimes, the nurturing provided by other members of the family has been sufficient for the development of a good, healthy, confident sense of self, and the child can break the silence immediately after the inception of the abuse (or prevent the abuse altogether). More often, the survivor endures the abuse and silence for quite a while.

Discovery and Disclosure of Incest

While the child may disclose to others about the abuse, it is usually after a long period of time, and may thus be dismissed as "lies," fantasy, or "past history" (i.e. "what's done is done"). Disclosure may occur accidentally or intentionally, while the survivor is still a child, or may not occur until some time after the abuse has stopped. Someone may witness the sexual abuse, unusual behavior may be questioned and then explained "accidentally," or the child may spontaneously disclose in response to genital infections, injury, or pregnancy. When disclosure is "accidental," responses to the child include crisis reactions and requests for immediate professional intervention.

If the child or the perpetrator uncovers the abuse intentionally (i.e. in order to terminate it), family members are likely to react with anger, anxiety, alarm, and shock, but crisis intervention may not be necessary. While survivors are usually responsible for terminating the abuse (through disclosure or threat), perpetrators have been known to "turn themselves in" in order to discontinue the abuse or to alleviate feelings of guilt, shame, deviance, or feared insanity.

After there has been a disclosure, those involved may wish to "forget" that their family has been stained by sexual abuse. Whether the disclosure was accidental or intentional, the family bonds together to suppress further discussion and action regarding the abuse. If the family *needs* the perpetrator, there will be even greater pressure to "just drop it." When this is the case, family members often conspire to coerce survivors to repress their memories, discontinue interventions and therapy, and cease vengeful or legal actions against the perpetrator.

Who Does It and To Whom?

Current research suggests that there are two types of incestuous families: chaotic and "normal-appearing." In both types of incested families, four preconditions must be met for sexual abuse to occur:

1) The potential perpetrator must want to abuse;
2) The potential perpetrator must overcome feelings of remorse, guilt, and shame which may prevent him/her from abusing;
3) The potential victim must be available, accessible, and easily isolated; and
4) The potential perpetrator must be able to manipulate the child so that the child will submit.

These family types will be summarized below. For more information, you may want to read *Child Sexual Abuse: New Theory & Research* by David Finklehor.

Chaotic Incested Families

Chaotic families in which incest occurs usually have the following characteristics:

- low socioeconomic status (i.e. lower income)
- limited education

- poor family functioning
- poor member functioning
- drug and alcohol abuse
- legal problems

Children are often left alone to take care of themselves and thus may be vulnerable to abuse by others (not only are they physically alone, but they feel empty and isolated). Members of chaotic families may be involved in multiple abuse, and younger siblings or children may learn to sexually abuse from parents and older siblings. If incest results in pregnancy, it is likely that the child will then be cared for within the incested family, and the incestuous patterns maintained. If survivors of chaotic families disclose, family members may or may not respond, but if justice is sought, the survivor from the chaotic family has a better chance of convicting her abuser than if he/she were raised in a "normal-appearing" family (not only does the perpetrator from the chaotic family have fewer resources with which to fight a legal battle, but the survivor from this family may be perceived as more "damaged" by the abuse than the survivor from a "normal-appearing" incested family, in which there may be less visible evidence of trauma). In contrast to the chaotic incested family described above is the "normal-appearing" family described below.

The "Normal-Appearing" Incested Family
The most common scenario in the "normal-appearing" family is one in which the perpetrator is the father and the survivor is his daughter or stepdaughter. These men can not be easily identified by race, religion, profession, age, socioeconomic status or relative intelligence. Just as their families appear normal on the outside, these offending fathers may also elude detection by others. Researchers have thus tried to categorize abusive fathers into specific "types," including symbiotic, psychopathic-sociopathic, pedophilic, and "other." As 80-85% of paternal perpetrators demonstrate symbiotic behavior, these profiles will be described in the Informational Highlights which follow. For further description and exemplification of these topologies, see the works of Justice and Justice or Courtois.

Fathers who abuse generally suffer from deep psychological distress, emotional immaturity, and isolation. Their sexual identities may be unclear, and they may not be able to communicate their sexual needs and desires to appropriate partners. In a quest for domination, or union with a submissive partner, the offending father often seeks out the weakest link in his family. A child's immaturity/vulnerability, coupled with a father's distorted thinking, can create a partnership ripe for sexual abuse.

Informational Highlight
The Symbiotic Introvert

Communication skills of the symbiotic introvert are generally limited, and he is often unable to identify and discuss his conflicts and issues with others (even those who may be able to assist him). He remains confused, distressed, angry, and isolated from his sources of support. This kind of abusive father often has very limited self-esteem, and feels powerless and inadequate. He may manipulate his daughter subtly—attempting to appear helpless or needy, rather than dominant or overpowering, in order to compel her to feel sorry for him. While you may find it hard to believe that a father could manipulate his own child in this way, abusive fathers often learned these patterns of behavior from their own sexually abusive parents or relatives.

Approximately 20% of these symbiotic abusers are symbiotic tyrants who manipulate others in order to feel dominant and powerful.

Informational Highlight
The Symbiotic Tyrant

These men often rely on physical force, and family members may live in fear of the tyrannical father. To the tyrant, women are a source of loyalty, submission, and sexual satisfaction, whether or not they are members of his family. The tyrant may be dominant and sadistic all of the time, or in particular situations, for instance, while under the influence of drugs or alcohol. Whether or not the tyrant uses physical force all of the time, or unpredictably, members of the family learn to fear and submit when in the presence of this kind of perpetrator.

Fathers who justify their abuse as "good" for their daughters are described as symbiotic rationalizers.

Informational Highlight
The Symbiotic Rationalizer

Rationalizations or excuses for the abuse that this kind of perpetrator uses may include:

- "My child seduced me"
- "I want to make sure that my child learns about sex the right way"
- "I just wanted to make my child feel good"
- "It was our special time together"
- "I'm keeping my family together by keeping my needs met at home"
- "I'm keeping our heritage pure by perpetuating my seed with my children"
- "I'm protecting my child from being 'molested' by others who may want her/him"

The most prominent characteristic of this kind of perpetrator is that he/she does not assume responsibility for harming or abusing the child or adolescent victim.

In addition to these ready-made rationalizations, the abusive father may learn to associate his child's body with his sexual fantasies. If he begins masturbating or sexually stimulating himself while fantasizing about the child, his sexual attraction to the child may increase. The combination of fantasy, with the excitement of risk-taking, fear of discovery, and distorted rationalization of the abuse, may heighten the perpetrator's abusive pleasure even further, thus perpetuating the sexual abuse.

Similar to others in dire circumstances, ten to fifty percent of these abusive fathers turn to alcohol, drugs or other escape routes in order to numb themselves to their inner turmoil, and/ or to mentally remove themselves from the pain they are causing others around them. Substance abuse frequently accompanies sexual abuse: in order for the offending father to meet his sexual and emotional needs with his daughter (without experiencing overwhelming guilt), he may have to mentally remove himself from the situation. As the survivor grows older, she herself may turn to drugs or alcohol: either to help her cope with further abuse or to shut out memories of past abuse. Often old images of abuse resurface when the survivor becomes sexually active or moves in with someone (even sharing living space with another person can remind the survivor of her incestuous home). The issue of survivors using drugs and alcohol in efforts to cope with abuse will be addressed in Chapter 3.

Additional Family Dynamics and Influences

Another factor that enables incest to occur is the role which the mother or other non-offending adult plays. Like the sexually abusive father, the non-offending mother is not differentiated by race, religion, profession, age, socioeconomic status or intelligence. Just as abusive fathers were described by "type," mothers can also be characterized. The three most common profiles for mothers are the dependent, care taking and submissive individuals. For a closer look at specific characteristics which comprise these "types," see works by Justice and Justice.

Mothers in incestuous families generally possess some typical characteristics. These include, but are not limited to:

- she appears weak or incapable to others
- she may appear to be emotionally distressed or handicapped

- she may believe that she can not financially support herself or family
- she is probably socially isolated and has a small network of friends and supportive others
- she is most likely unavailable to her children, because of her emotional state, attention to the perpetrator, or activities outside the home
- she has low self-esteem, probably feels intimidated by the perpetrator, and feels worthless as a parent, wife, and woman
- she is likely to be a survivor of sexual abuse

In her "weakened" state, the mother in an incestuous family may encourage her children to assume responsibilities that she feels she can no longer manage, facilitating the parentification of one or all of the children.

Informational Highlight
The Parentified Child

When parents feel incompetent, unable or handicapped in some way, they may demand that their children take on responsibilities for which the children are unprepared. Those responsibilities may include:

- child care
- daily household chores
- provision of emotional support
- acting as confidante and mediator
- sexual gratification of the spouse

While it is healthy for children to learn to handle some responsibility, in incestuous families the responsibilities expected to be managed by the children far exceed their resources and coping abilities. The most prominent transgression in incestuous families is the misplaced responsibility of the daughter to satisfy her father's sexual and emotional needs.

When incest is finally disclosed, the mother may or may not believe her daughter. While some mothers have sensed that something was happening between father and daughter, others deny any knowledge of the abuse. Frequently the mother becomes immobilized by the disclosure, and even though she may want to be supportive to her daughter, she will struggle as she sorts through a myriad of feelings:

- Anger at her husband
  "How could you do this to my child?"
- Anger at her daughter
  "Why didn't you confide in me?"
- Guilt
  "It's my fault that this has happened!"
- Betrayal by her husband
  "How could you do this to our marriage?"
- Betrayal by her daughter
  "How could you keep the incest a secret?"
- Hatred
  "You've hurt my child and you've hurt us! Look at what you've done!"
- Repulsion
  "You must be a monster for touching my child in a sexual way!"
- Jealousy of her daughter
  "How come he gave you special attention when he wouldn't even attend to me?"
- Confusion
  "I love the man I married, but I can't love him if I'm going to support my daughter through this."
- Failure
  "How can I be a mother if I let all this happen?"

Just as there are some typical characteristics for the fathers who abuse their daughters and the mothers who fail to protect, there are typical characteristics for the daughters who survive such incest. Incest survivors are frequently the eldest child in the family, though the abuser may also violate younger children concurrently or subsequently. If sexual abuse occurs prior to age five, the survivor may be unable to mentally comprehend what these sexual "games" mean, and as a result may not experience shame or guilt, but instead may become prematurely "eroticized" by her father. If the child experiences the contact as traumatic, abusive, and "wrong," she will likely feel shame, guilt, and fear and may use very basic coping strategies such as repression and denial in order to manage the physical and emotional situation. As the sexual abuse continues, the daughter becomes parentified and sexualized, and may assume other responsibilities that are normally held by adults in the family. Survivors commonly submit in these households until they are physically able to flee—to marriage or independence.

In addition to the description provided in this chapter of the typical father-daughter incest, there are further detailed descriptions of the parents, siblings, and relatives who sexually abuse family members in many of the books listed in Chapter 10.

You've just spent a great deal of time trying to take in information about the "typical" kinds of sexual abuse. In order to digest this material, try the following exercises.

Exercise #1: "What I've learned so far..."

Take out a piece of paper and a pen (or an audio cassette and tape recorder if you prefer) and make notes of what you've learned so far about your partner. Write or record for at least ten minutes, no matter how confused you may be about the material.

Exercise #2: "The questions I still have..."

After you've completed Exercise #1, reread what you have written or listen to what you have recorded. Now make a list of questions you have about your partner and the things you would like to learn. Refer to this list as you read on. It will help you stay focused on what's important to you!

Prognosis:
What does all of this mean for you and your partner?

Recovery from child and adolescent sexual abuse requires great strength and commitment not only from the survivor but also from you, the partner. Healing can provide the greatest rewards, but it can be a painful and confusing process. During the initial stages of healing, a caring and nurturing relationship between partners can make all the difference in the world. Relationships at this stage must withstand the vigor of the "psychic surgery," required to reduce the emotional scars left by the sexual abuse.

If this chapter has given you some information and insight into the problem of child sexual abuse, then you are already more informed than a large percentage of the population. And if that is all you gain from reading this chapter, then you have achieved a lot. If you were able to more clearly understand your partner or to better empathize with him/her as a result of your efforts, then you have given yourself and your partner an invaluable gift. Read on and you may experience more benefits.

Chapter 2
Scars and Symptoms

How is the Survivor Affected By the Abuse?
Children who endure sexual abuse of any kind are an unusual breed. While some children cope with their abuse through physical or mental illness, there are a great many children who simply cordon off the abused area of their lives and develop a facade, alternative personae, alter ego, or superhero image, to manage the abuse so that they can continue to function in other areas of their lives. While these children experience great distress and fear when they are abused, they may continue to function quite capably in school and at home. Shelly recalls the facade she developed as a child:

> *My father was in the military while I was growing up, so we moved around a lot. And since I was the eldest of six kids, it was up to me to make sure that everyone was getting along OK in school and all, and that no one was getting beaten up at lunch or anything. When my dad started molesting me, I was only ten, but I didn't let that mess me up. I just added it to my other responsibilities: now I was daughter, sister, tutor, baby-sitter, cook, housekeeper, confidante and wife.*

Even though children who have been abused may be able to develop "false selves" to manage the tasks and expectations of daily life, the sexually abused child lives in fear: haunted by memories and flashbacks of abuse he/she has already suffered, terrified that someone will discover the abuse that has already occurred, and petrified that the abuse will be perpetuated into the future. When the child is being abused by a family member, or a close friend of the family (whose interaction with the child is predictable and/or frequent), the child may become even more distressed. When a relative or family friend abuses a child, the child learns that adults may not be trustworthy, and he/she may have difficulty with trust in future relationships. When the non-offending parent or relative fails to respond or to protect the child in the abusive situation, trust may be impaired further.

While children who survive sexual abuse may continue to function fairly well in some settings, it is common for the child's behavior to change after the inception of the abuse (behavioral change ranges in quality, duration and onset among children). Dr. Christine Courtois estimates that approximately twenty to forty percent of abused children show pathological signs and symptoms immediately following the onset of the abuse.

Informational Highlight
Common signs of sexual abuse in children

Some common signs displayed by children who have survived sexual abuse include but are not limited to:
- social withdrawal
- regression to more infantile behavior (e.g. thumb sucking or clinging)
- agitation, hyperactivity, aggression toward others
- loss of appetite
- nightmares, insomnia, frequent waking, and sleepwalking
- bed wetting and fecal soiling
- frequent gagging and dry heaving in children and adolescents or spitting in toddlers and infants
- explicit sexual knowledge, behavior, or language unusual for their age, including excessive masturbation and promiscuity
- frequent genital infections and sexually transmitted diseases

These symptoms or signs may persist or they may be replaced by other responses over time. Impacts of the abuse may be manifested emotionally, psychologically, and/or behaviorally. In addition, signs and symptoms that are often observed in older children and adolescents are noted in the following Informational Highlight.

Informational Highlight

Symptoms of older children and adolescent survivors

Some of the behaviors often seen in older children, adolescents and adults who have been sexually abused include:
- recurrent physical complaints
  - infections, abdominal and/or genital pain, muscle aches, severe headaches, and dizziness
- eating disorders and/or sudden weight gain/loss
- addiction
  - chemical, food, gambling, or sex
- severe startle response
  - flinching, crying, or "paralysis" when touched by another
- overly seductive behavior
  - promiscuity to prostitution
- sexual problems and aversions
- social isolation
- changed sensitivity to the environment
- hypervigilance or hypovigilance
- "clumsiness," always bumping into furniture and people as he/she is unaware of his/her body
- change in school or work performance
- workaholism
- parentification or excessive responsibility-taking
- delinquency
  - lying, stealing, truancy, and running away
- religiosity
- self-harm
  - self-inflicted bruising, breaking of bones, cutting, burning, tattooing, piercing, and suicide attempts

Physical Symptoms of Sexual Abuse

A number of the physical complaints described by survivors of sexual abuse correspond to the symptoms associated with somatization, such as abdominal and/or genital pain, muscle aches, and dizziness. Frequently survivors do not know how to express their feelings directly and thus express their painful feelings through their bodies, so that they and others can respond to the survivor's needs for nurturing and protection, without recognizing the true source of the survivor's pain (which might cause the survivor to feel exposed, vulnerable, and humiliated). Somatization is explained more fully in Chapter 3.

A unique form of somatization that occurs as the survivor is beginning to "pop" memories of long-forgotten sexual abuse is the body memory. Body memories are intrusive, overwhelming physical signs that the individual has experienced trauma at an earlier time which take the place of visual or auditory memories. This stimulation may be experienced as pervasive physical "electricity" in the entire body, but is more frequently site-specific. Most survivors experience body memories prior to the attainment of any visual memories of the abuse, but some survivors receive memories from many sensory sources at once. Some research indicates that body memories are most frequently experienced by those who were abused at an age prior to the development of complex language (e.g. age two or three).

Body memories, or the tactile impression that one is being impacted or touched by another human being or object, are usually extremely frightening and may render the survivor helpless to the primitive messages being sent through her/his body. Because you are close to the survivor, it is likely that you will be with your partner if she/he does have a body memory. If this should happen, it will be important for you to assure your partner that he/she is not crazy and that the experience will be temporary. Above all, don't let your partner "forget" where or who she/he is, or who you are) and keep your partner free of physical harm.

Research suggests that these physical symptoms of early trauma may be "abuse site-specific" or can reflect a more generalized physical distress. Abuse to the breasts, thighs, buttocks, genitals, and genitourinary organs frequently leaves the survivor with chronic pain, infection, fears, phobias, and anxieties about these areas. Remnants of abusive or incestuous oral sex may be manifested as nausea, gagging, vomiting, choking, and spitting responses to chewing, swallowing, and oral exams (i.e. in the dentist's office). Dr. Courtois suggests that "rectal discomfort, pain, hemorrhoids, constipation and diarrhea are associated with anal intercourse, enemas, and anal-lingus." More generalized physical symptoms include:

- gastrointestinal problems
- severe menstrual pain
- pain during intercourse
- skin irritations
- muscular tension
- migraines
- high blood pressure
- fixated joints (especially the hips)
- ringing in the ears.

Behavioral Signs of Sexual Abuse

While most of the addictions are described as coping strategies in Chapter 3, they can also be considered behavioral effects of sexual abuse. After being abused, many survivors turn to chemicals, food and gambling, to drive the memories away, and to numb themselves to the events of the past. Survivors may also develop sexual addiction, which may be manifested as behaviors ranging from promiscuity to prostitution. Ann describes her addiction below:

> After Gary abused me, I felt so weird. I was so confused. I didn't understand what had happened to me. You know, I was a good girl, raised Catholic, and of course, I hadn't had sex or anything before I met Gary, and after that happened, I began to wonder what I was good for. I blamed myself for what he'd done, and I kind of began to think of myself as "a lay." I was with everyone after that. I remember one time, at a dance, I was taking two or three guys an hour into the guys' locker room. You know, I still don't remember much about what happened then... I guess I just spaced out and let them do what they wanted to. It didn't matter, because to me, I was doing what I was meant for. To me, having sex that way at least allowed me to feel like I was in control. I called the shots rather than some guy. Only trouble was, I had to call the shots as often as I could, because otherwise the pain, and violation, and helplessness of my abuse might leak through: sex became a necessity.

While other survivors have relied on chemicals or psychological defenses, Ann demonstrates how her use of sex helped her maintain her sense of control over overwhelming feelings of helplessness. It is important to note that it was not Ann's desire for sexual interaction which enabled her to maintain a fleeting sense of composure, but her need for absolute control over this aspect of her existence that enabled her to contain her feelings of pain, violation and helplessness. For more information on sexual addiction, read *Out of the Shadows* and *Don't Call it Love* by Patrick Carnes.

Other survivors seek out sexually-dominated or abusive relationships not only to control sexuality and sexual interaction, but also to master this particular kind of relationship. A fairly common example of the effects of this kind of involvement is the Battered Spouse Syndrome, in which a spouse who has been abused (by the spouse or by another perpetrator) may remain in the relationship because he/she believes that, "Next time it will be different." The spouse may also fantasize about stopping the abuse and developing a more satisfying relationship with the perpetrator. Unfortunately, it is rare that the survivor ever masters the abusive relationship because in order to do so the abusive individual must either change his/her pattern of responding to others (which is possible but unlikely in many situations), or submit to the survivor. When submission becomes the goal of the relationship, a survivor becomes a perpetrator and the vicious circle is perpetuated. In addition to spouses who remain in battering relationships because of the desire to master the abusive relationship, there are spouses who remain in violent marriages because they feel incapable of leaving. Many are without financial and emotional resources to leave.

Another impact of sexual abuse (which can also be identified in the Battered Spouse Syndrome) is the inability or failure of the survivor to make and maintain personal boundaries. When the abuse is committed, the individual learns that the personal boundaries that he/she has set may not be respected by others. Even the very primitive boundaries that an individual sets by donning clothing can be broken by the perpetrator who decides that he/she can place his/her hands underneath that clothing against a victim's will. Other violations of personal boundaries include but are not limited to:

- Disrespect for privacy
  - Examples:
  1) a stepfather who repeatedly enters the bathroom while his stepdaughter or stepson is bathing
  2) a mother who demands to know about every aspect of her son's school day, especially the deeply personal information
- The encroachment of an individual's personal space
  - Example:
  when the abuser "gets in your face"
- The invasion of personal boundaries
  - Example:
  physical abuse

Once the survivor recognizes that her/his personal boundaries are not respected by others, self-respect may diminish drastically, and the survivor may no longer attempt to maintain those boundaries. Gail tells her story:

My step-dad was a drunk, and the drunker he got, the meaner he got. That's when he was most likely to rape me. And, when I could see it coming, I'd sneak out. Sometimes, I'd be doing my homework, and not really be aware of how many scotches he'd tossed back and that was when I was really in trouble. Then he'd come over and get into my face and start taunting me about how I thought I was so much better than him, because I was going to go to college. He really liked to demean me, and raping me was the worst degradation that he could make me experience.

After a while, I stopped experiencing the massive feelings of invasion when he'd get into my face, or push me around. And I lost that sense of body awareness that most people have when they're in crowds. I remember going to school, and getting jostled around and pushed about during the change of classes, and not even feeling the sensation of my body being touched by other

*bodies. I just didn't even consciously experience
the physical invasion, because I didn't have
boundaries to violate anymore. But psychologically, I imprinted it all, and it's taken me years
to get back that sense of my positive, physical
self.*

In this vignette, Gail became hypovigilant as a result of
repeated violations of her personal boundaries. She lost her
sense of what was happening about and to her. Some survivors
become even more disoriented than Gail, and come to rely on a
cloak of chaos, whereby the survivor learns to thrive in the
chaotic environment, as the crazy feelings inside are matched
by the external disarray, creating a sense of normalcy for the
survivor. Still other survivors experience the opposite effect after
being sexually abused: these individuals become hypervigilant,
or extremely sensitive to all aspects of their environments. Laura
(whose comments are located in a vignette at the beginning of
Chapter 3) experienced hypervigilance about the shower in her
home, while Katherine (whose comments appear below)
experienced a more pervasive hypervigilance. Katherine recalls
feeling inundated by stimuli after she remembered her molest:

*After I remembered, I felt like I was hot-wired.
Every nerve in my body worked overtime. I'd be
sitting in my room, trying to relax, you know, and
the dog would walk into the room, and I'd jump
about six feet in the air! Every noise in the house
felt like it was blasting inside my head, and scared
me to death. I had to know where every door and
window was, and whether it was locked or not. I
needed to know what everyone was doing and
where they were. I needed to know everything
about everything in order to feel like the world
wasn't going to come crashing in on me.*

Other survivors mold their hypervigilance into a honed
intuition. The survivor with this ability is likely to help others,
as a therapist or customer service representative, for instance.
In these occupations, the survivor can employ his/her intuition
adaptively, to assist others, and may be experienced as quite
understanding and supportive (e.g. the client who notes that

the survivor, "always seems to know just what I'm thinking and feeling!"). Even though the survivor may come to use hypervigilance adaptively, it is important that he/she take care not to rely on this method too heavily. Hypervigilance, in any form, can enable the survivor to avoid feeling or emoting at all.

Given the amount of energy consumed by daily survival following sexual abuse, especially if the survivor is using drugs or alcohol to cope, it seems logical that performance at work or school will diminish in quality. Yet, while you might expect a performance "slide" as a sign of distress, you might not have guessed that your partner's grades or production could have increased after the abuse. This phenomena can be described as performance par excellence, and can just as surely be an effect of abuse as is a downhill slide. Survivors who functioned better at work or school after being abused may have become accustomed to throwing themselves into work, probably to avoid distressing feelings, thoughts, and memories. Unfortunately, this over functioning can have disastrous long-term effects, as survivors feel less and less connected to their work products and processes, and begin to experience the effects of stress on functioning. Ginger described her workaholism as a necessity after she was raped.

> *I just wanted to lie around the apartment all day. Didn't want to go out, to go to work, to shop, even to breathe fresh air. I didn't want the world to see what Jim had done to me. Several days after the rape, I decided to check in with work, via my home computer modem. And after I read my electronic mail, I figured I'd just respond with a few memos. Hours later, I realized how good, and how productive I felt. I looked over the work I'd completed and I felt proud, and able. I could do this, if only this, and no one, not even Jim, could take it away from me. This product was mine, and there in the document, I was in control. And that was when I knew I needed to work more, and that I'd do everything I could to continue working, whatever the cost.*

While the coping behavior of these individuals is less obvious to the observer (i.e. it may not be readily interpreted by others as coping, but instead as increased productivity), it is reflective of inner turmoil just as much as is chemical addiction. The key to identification of these coping behaviors lies in change.

Other behaviors that may change in intensity or frequency as a result of sexual abuse include lying, stealing, and truancy. Often administrators, parents, or partners interpret a combination of these behaviors as delinquency, sociopathic, or as an impulse disorder. Observers and supporters may fail to see the adaptive qualities that these behaviors may have for a survivor. Yet, not only do these behaviors have an indirect value, as attention is directed toward a survivor (so that he/she can receive some assistance, even if it is for an unrelated incident), some of the behaviors, such as lying, become a necessity for a survivor. Emily recalls lying as a child, during and after the duration of her incest experiences.

> At first, I had to lie to cover up for my dad. My mom would ask him, 'Were you in Em's room last night?' And I would pipe up, 'Oh, no, Mom, I saw Dad watching a football game real late.' It was better if I lied, because then Dad would love me more. I figured he'd stop when I asked him to then. But he didn't. Then I had to lie when the guidance counselor asked me if I was having problems at home, when I started failing classes. What was I going to say? I could never tell on my Dad, he would never forgive me. Then I had to learn to lie to myself as I grew older. I couldn't tolerate the reality of the incest, so I tried to pretend that it never happened. But it did, and I couldn't lie well enough to hide it from myself.

If the survivor does not receive needed assistance with more "lightweight" tactics, he/she may use more extreme coping strategies. The young abuse survivor may try to run away from home if the perpetrator is a member of the household. Adult survivors may continue running, even years later, not specifically from the residence of perpetrators, but because they have used this technique successfully in the past. Many survivors believe that "if they can't catch you, they can't hurt you." Unfortunately, if others can't "catch" you, they can't help you either.

Sometimes, survivors do not flee physically, but they may isolate themselves socially and emotionally from others. This withdrawal may be limited or may be more comprehensive, depending on experiences of the survivor. Some female survivors who have been abused by men find that they cannot be within ten feet of men after experiencing violations, but they may gain pleasure and sustenance from female interaction. Other survivors find that they cannot endure the company of anyone. Of these survivors, some fear that others will take advantage of their vulnerability; that those who are close can "see the damage"; and/or that those who interact with them will be "soiled" through any association. These survivors, who need support of peers and resource providers, are left to fend for themselves at a time when isolation may only help to maintain the emotional damage caused by abuse.

There are also other forms of isolation which are more subtle to detect. Ginger's workaholism allowed her to feel productive, but also kept her bound to the safety of her computer terminal. Another coping strategy similar to workaholism is religiosity, or an increased use of religion to manage thoughts, feelings and memories. In many situations, religion can provide comfort and safety unavailable elsewhere for the survivor. But in other cases, religion is used to distance from others who may otherwise be effective resources. In addition, when religion is used to negate, detach, or avoid the abused part of the self, the survivor can become emotionally disabled and stunted.

Frank, who was abused by his maternal grandmother as a child, first tried to manage his pain through alcohol, food, and sex. He entered therapy and began to experience the full impact of his emotional pain as he worked through his sexual abuse. But after becoming involved with a religious organization, Frank left therapy, claiming that the church focused "only on the positive, and that emphasis on the negative events of (his) past life would only increase (his) spiritual sickness." While his religiosity may help Frank recover from the effects of his sexual abuse, it is likely that his repressed pain will reemerge at a later date.

Some of the impacts of sexual abuse are even more extreme than addiction, workaholism, and religiosity. Those survivors who rely on more primitive psychological coping strategies may self-mutilate or attempt suicide. After Evan raped Blanca, she became very self-destructive. Since Blanca was raped by her sister's husband, Blanca found that her biggest source of support, Mira, was not available to her. Blanca relates some of her story below:

> *When I was finally safe, you know, I realized how badly Evan had hurt me. But I could only think how much I needed to talk to Mira, but I couldn't talk to Mira. I could never tell Mira that Evan and I had sex. And the more I thought about it, the worse I felt about myself for going over there, for getting high, for hurting Mira. I wanted to hurt myself then, so I burned myself with cigarettes. But that didn't help, and it didn't make the pain go away. I tried to convince myself that nothing had happened, but then I began to feel pretty unreal myself. I cut myself then, to find out if I was real... My blood was sure real enough, so I figured I couldn't pretend anymore. I didn't know what to do, and it hurt so bad, I figured I'd end it all. I took a load of pills, but lucky me, it didn't work. Three years later, after several abusive relationships, and being raped a number of times, I finally got myself into counseling. It never occurred to me before how much I wanted to hurt Evan, and even Mira, for what had happened. I just didn't know how to express that. Instead of hurting them, I just hurt myself, over and over again. And the reason it still hurt so bad, is 'cuz I wasn't hurtin' the right person!*

In her own way, Blanca grasps a significant concept for survivors: that pain and rage are often turned inwards, and expressed as self-destruction and self-mutilation, when the survivor fears more direct expression of these emotions. During the recovery process, survivors learn how to express these emotions actively and directly, and generally feel less need for self-destructive behaviors.

Informational Highlight
Self-injury

Self-injury may include but is not limited to the following self-induced behaviors and actions:

- body piercing
- body "pricking" or "needling" (e.g. with safety or straight pins)
- body carving and cutting
- picking at skin repeatedly so that self-induced wounds cannot heal
- body burning (e.g. with matches or cigarettes)
- body bruising or flagellating
- forced penetration of objects into the mouth, vagina or anus
- ingestion of poisons or toxins
- binding body parts perceived as "dirty" or "evil"

Some survivors become addicted to self-harm and they may resist letting go of this coping strategy. They may actually experience a "high" after cutting, burning, or otherwise damaging their bodies. In addition to the indirect expression of anger, self-injury may be perceived as soothing to some survivors who have come to associate physical pain with attention, comfort, and self-worth. Survivors may also self-mutilate when they believe that they have made an error and must be punished. In order to better understand this destructive behavior in yourself or your partner, it is important that you determine what purpose the self-harm serves.

Emotional Symptoms of Sexual Abuse
In addition to the ways in which sexual abuse impacts behavior, survivors are often affected emotionally. Some emotions experienced frequently by survivors include:
- anxiety
- anger
- fear
  - of those who have or may hurt them

- that they are insane
- of failure
- of success
- shame
- guilt
- confusion
- restricted or overwhelming emotions
- powerlessness
- a sense of being different from others
- betrayal
  - by offending and non-offending adults
  - by their own bodies for response to sexual stimulation
- isolation
- worthlessness
- humiliation
- self-hatred
  - of self
  - of one's genitalia
- depression
- suicidal impulses

Suzanne's isolation, differences, and shame are reflected with poignancy in her story below:

I remember the first time I told anyone about my abuse. It seems so clear to me even now: I was a sophomore in high school, and kind of a lonely time for me, as my boyfriend had gone away to college, and I had only a few friends. Among them were two brothers, John and Stan. The three of us spent a lot of time together, both working and playing.

The three of us signed up with about fifteen other students to be trained as peer counselors. The program provided a year's worth of training, after which we would serve on counseling teams. During that first year together, we were given the opportunity to get to know one another, and to get to know ourselves better. One of the vehicles for that process was a support group, where we discussed our experiences.

At one of our first meetings, Pat, our group facilitator, asked us to think about what made us the way we were, then asked for volunteers to share. I was sitting across from Pat, and Stan and John were to my immediate left, and Sandy sat to their left. Beatrice was to my right, then Mary, then Steve, and the rest are now a blur. Ever since I can remember, I've always volunteered to be first in groups, so that my turn can be over, and I can "enjoy" the rest of the experience. And, when Pat posed her question to us, my insides began to turn upside down, and I felt as if I might pass out. I knew what I wanted to share with my peers, but knew that I'd faint or throw up if I didn't do it quickly. I was so terrified, my heart pounded in chest, and I could feel the burning in my cheeks before I even began to speak. I started tentatively, trying to ease myself into my "confession" with vague words, and I remember hearing myself say, "I am who I am because of what happened to me a long time ago." I continued, and forced myself to say that I had been "accosted" at age six by a friend of the family. As the words came tumbling out of my mouth, I saw Stan's head drop softly to his hands, placed gently on his knees, and heard the barely audible "oh, God" from not only his lips, but from those of the others around me.

As I recall the incident now, I sense that my peers were trying in their way to empathize with me, but what I experienced then was the horror of the moment, and ensuing shame for finally breaking my silence. My sense of self was saved only by my own reminder of my survival, and the reassuring words of Pat, who disclosed that her daughter had been gang-raped at age eight. I had wished for the deep empathy and support of my peers, but found only maternal arms to hold me.

These feelings and experiences may often be associated with difficulties with the following:

- feeling positive
  - self-love and nurturing
  - self-enjoyment
  - self-esteem
- feeling successful
  - motivation
  - achievement
  - perfectionism
- feeling safe with others
  - self-protection
  - trust (in self, intuition, others)
- "fitting-in" or intimate relationships
  - no role models for healthy relationships or affection
  - relationships with inappropriate or abusive partners
  - repeated testing of partners and their loyalty and love
- healthy sexuality
  - lack of sexual desire or pleasure
  - compulsive sexual activity or inactivity
  - desire for total control during sex
  - problems with staying "tuned in" during sex
  - inability to say no to sexual requests or demands
  - using sex as a means to attain nurturing or other emotional needs
  - using others or being used by others for sexual exploitation
  - flashbacks during sex

Issues of sexuality and relationships are discussed more fully in Chapters 4 through 7.

All of your partner's feelings which have not yet been expressed or explored inhibit his or her regeneration of self-love, self-nurturing, self-enjoyment, self-worth, and self-esteem. These feelings, common for abuse survivors, create great emotional obstacles to the growth and development of the inner self.

In order for the survivor to heal, he/she must be able to identify the feelings which are associated with the abuse and break the silence: your partner must share with you and others the painful feelings of anger, shame, guilt, fear, isolation, and humiliation stemming from the abuse. The identification and expression of these feelings can enable your partner to gain control over emotions which may have previously "propelled" the survivor regardless of his/her desires or ambitions. Survivors often notice a reduction in feelings of self-hatred, deprecation, depression, and suicidal feelings accompanying the release of these suppressed emotions.

When an individual is abused, his/her sense of self-worth is damaged immensely. A survivor may experience feelings of shame, guilt, confusion, powerlessness, worthlessness, humiliation or depression—as signs of weakness and vulnerability that will deter others from treating the survivor with respect and kindness. And, since others have already responded to the survivor abusively, your partner may believe that he/she does not deserve more humane treatment.

Because your partner may not feel in control of his/her emotions (or may feel so different from others or may feel uncomfortable around others), he/she may feel incapable of developing healthy relationships. In addition, because the survivor has a limited sense of self-worth, he/she may actually select an abusive partner. These partners may even resemble the original abuser and may disrespect, disregard, manipulate, and abuse the survivor. While your partner may not have consciously chosen an abusive relationship, he/she may have fallen back on this type of relationship because of low self-worth caused by circumstances, events, or memories of past abuse.

The survivor's ability to succeed and prosper is also restricted by low self-worth. Often, sexual abuse survivors see themselves as "losers" or "damaged goods," and this wounded sense of self impairs the survivor's ability to perceive personal strengths and valued qualities. When your partner is unable to see his/her strengths, he/she may develop problems of motivation and fear of failure. If your partner is afraid that others can see his/her weaknesses, he/she may try harder to overcompensate to prevent ever feeling vulnerable again.

Often, it is important that the sexual abuse survivor "understand" what has happened. Children frequently make up explanations for what has happened because the alternative is unthinkable: that a trusted adult has intentionally harmed them, and has violated their boundaries and rights to human decency. Adolescents and adults are less likely to rewrite history, even when they do not pop memories of abuse until much later. The truth is remembered but the effects are the same: trust in self and others is nearly destroyed.

Sexual abuse leaves the survivor feeling that he/she has nowhere to turn, inward or outward. When faced with ultimate violation by another human being, he/she has been unable to protect himself/herself. While the survivor may have been able to psychologically shutdown to endure the abuse, he/she was unable to escape the attack. The survivor may feel as if he/she cannot trust him/herself to keep danger at arm's length. Past experience of being unable to protect one's self, coupled with feelings of confusion and fear (that one is insane because this can't have actually happened!), emotional liability, powerlessness, deviance, self-hatred (of self and of one's genitalia), and suicidal tendency may prevent the survivor from trusting her/his instincts or intuition for years following the abuse.

This lack of self-trust may be reflected in the survivor's inability to make even minor decisions (e.g. what clothes to wear to work) without frequent feedback from others. Your partner may even learn to tune out his/her internal signals entirely and opt to listen to the advice of others exclusively. Unfortunately, when this happens, the survivor can be vulnerable to manipulation by others who use the survivor's gullibility to get what they want.

In addition to feeling that he/she may be unable to completely trust him/herself, the survivor is likely to experience feelings of anger, fear, and betrayal after being abused. As a result, it is likely that the survivor may experience a distrust of others, especially those with the same qualities or characteristics as the perpetrator. When your partner is feeling frightened or distrustful, he/she may isolate, strongly assert his/her independence, or enroll in self-defense or martial arts courses.

As you may have noticed, issues of trust become even more complicated in an intimate relationship. When your partner feels that he/she cannot trust you, he/she shuts off a part of himself/herself. The survivor may be unwilling to be vulnerable and to share openly with you, decreasing the degree of intimacy that can develop between you. Issues of trust, commitment, repeated testing of your loyalty and love, and conflicts regarding sexuality may appear shortly after the inception of the relationship. These issues will be addressed more fully in Chapter 5.

Finally, as mentioned above, survivors may face a number of problems associated with sensuality and sexuality—beyond the issues elicited during a love relationship. Conflicts of sensuality revolve around the individual's physical appearance and feelings about being perceived as a sexual being. Conflicts around sexuality focus on the gender of the survivor, the acceptance of his/her genitalia, sexual preference, ability to engage in sexual relationships, the breadth and complexity of those relationships, and the manner in which sexuality is explored. These issues are addressed in Chapter 4.

Psychological Effects of Sexual Abuse

In addition to the impacts which child sexual abuse may have on behavior and emotion, there may be extensive psychological effects. These may include but are not limited to:

- poor memory and concentration
- psychological fragmentation
  - "I feel like I'm coming apart at the seams"
- the tendency for dissociation
  - "spacing out"
- a need and/or demand for absolute control in areas not associated with the abuse
- changed sensitivity to the environment
  - a need or desire for a "cloak of chaos"
  - hypervigilance or hypovigilance
- mental illness

Many effects of sexual abuse also act as coping strategies. These psychological processes are further addressed in Chapter 3.

In addition to these behavioral, emotional and psychological signs and symptoms of sexual abuse, Eliana Gil has outlined a number of roles which allow the survivor to manage his/her memories and experiences associated with abuse. These will be summarized for you; however, you may also want to read Gil's books, *Outgrowing the Pain* and *Outgrowing the Pain Together* for further information. The roles may be characterized by caretaking or rescuing; by hiding ("lost souls"); by demonstration of "tough guy" behavior; and by the emotional explosiveness of the "walking time-bomb."

Informational Highlight
Survivors who caretake

___

The caretaking role allows the survivor to provide the kind of unconditional love, attention, and nurturing that he/she never received as an abused child or adolescent. Through giving, the survivor believes that he/she will finally experience at least one part of the giving/receiving equation. While it may seem easier for the survivor to ask others to provide love and nurturing, this experience might be too frightening. After all, the survivor would have to expose that vulnerable part of himself/herself which needs such loving care. The survivor works at giving, probably to feel better about himself/herself. Unfortunately, when others do not give in return, an unconscious resentment begins to develop within the survivor (no matter how much he/she denies it). The development of nurturing and love must be mutually inclusive, and it requires both giving and receiving. If your partner has been doing all of the nurturing in your relationship, you might want to encourage him/her to relax a little, and let you take care of him/her for a while.

___

Yvonne reflects on her career as a guidance counselor and "caretaker":

> *You know, I thought all my life that I wanted to give other kids the kind of treatment that I just didn't get when I was growing up. I just wanted someone to listen to me, and to say, "Hey, are you OK? Is something wrong?" So that I wouldn't have to rip my heart open on my own to expose my traumas. So I thought, what better way to do that than to return to that stage of life and make things different. So now I work in the high school, seeing kids all day long, trying to listen hard, and to give them tender care. It feels good to be hearing the words that I wanted to hear, coming out of*

my mouth. You know, I try so hard, but sometimes, these kids just don't change. They stay with the boyfriend who hits them, or cut classes even when they know that negative attention isn't what they need. That's when I feel like I'm not making a difference, and that this maybe wasn't the best idea.

While Yvonne has a good grasp on what is important to her, she doesn't recognize the negative impacts of her co-dependency. Yvonne is still giving because she wants others to feel good, and her self-esteem relies on changes made by others, rather than on events and processes over which she has control. Yvonne's career will not bring her emotional satisfaction until she learns to do the job for herself. Yvonne must learn to generate her own esteem and self-worth based on her value as a human being.

Other survivors may manage their sexual abuse experiences by taking on the role of the "lost soul."

Informational Highlight
"Lost souls"

Lost souls may hide with their physical characteristics, behavior, and personalities. They hide behind glasses, layers of fat or androgynous thinness, loose and formless clothing, and cosmetics. They hide so that they will not be noticed because in the past being singled out has resulted in physical, emotional and psychological trauma.

While hiding may be sufficient for some survivors, others may need to drift endlessly in order to maintain their secrecy. They may not only hide behind physical and behavioral qualities, but they may wander from place to place, connecting with no one, failing to set down roots anywhere, so that they can remain safe in their anonymity.

Similar to those who hide are other survivors who present themselves as "tough guys." While this term may conjure up images of leather-jacketed hoodlums (and may, in fact, include these characters), the presentation may not nearly be as strong as that. Review the Informational Highlight for further description of the "tough guys."

Informational Highlight
"Tough guys"

How many times has your partner had a bad day, or injured him/herself, and when asked if he/she needed anything the response was, "Oh, no, I'm just fine. Go on with whatever you were doing." This is usually tough guy behavior. In this situation, your partner is hiding his/her true feelings (e.g. "I feel bad!," "I really need you to come here and take care of me!," "I'm so unhappy that I could just die!"), in order to cover his/her vulnerabilities to avoid being hurt further. This creates a nearly impossible situation because the survivor needs attention and nurturing but is often unwilling to be vulnerable enough to ask for his/her needs to be met directly. Unless you become a good mind-reader, your partner will need to learn to trust you enough to expose his/her needs so that you can help meet those needs as they arise.

Quite markedly different from tough guy behavior is that of the emotionally labile "walking time bomb."

Informational Highlight

"Walking time-bombs"

These survivors actively emote, especially angry or resentful feelings. They manage their experience of sexual abuse through active self-protection. For example, the survivor who fears that his girlfriend will leave him, leaves her first, just to avoid the pain she might cause him. While other survivors may use their anger constructively (e.g. the surviving attorney who fights for children's rights in sexual abuse cases), the emotional ability of these "time bombs" works destructively (i.e. against the survivor).

Tom, who fits all characteristics of the "walking time-bomb," recalls how his anger erupted in a bar fight.

> *I was sitting at the bar... and a woman was sitting at the other end, and damned if she doesn't look like my mom. I mean, she had darker hair and her nose was bigger, but she sure reminded me of my mom. I know it's not polite to stare, so I keep looking into my beer, and all these feelings start coming up. I got so angry about what my mom did to me, and all of the sudden I had to get it out. I just couldn't stand the way she was making me feel. I start listening to these to guys next to me at the bar, talking about sports, and as soon as I see my opening, I goad the one guy about his football pick for the week. Well, this guy gets on my case and says, "Who the hell are you anyway" and all, and I just hauled off and hit him. Then he hit me, then these other two guys got into it, and well, you know. It felt so good, and the more I fought, the less angry I was about what happened when I was a kid, until finally I just couldn't feel anything anymore. I think that's when the cops arrived.*

Tom seems to recognize pretty clearly how he chose to express his historical angry feelings through physical aggression. The problem is that violence is not a socially acceptable strategy for coping with emotions. It is important that Tom find a vehicle for releasing his emotions in a more productive and constructive, rather than destructive, manner.

Not all survivors cope with their sexual abuse experiences in the same way, and not all assume clearly-defined roles. But the survivor manages the pain of abuse in some way. As a partner, you must learn to "read" your partner and learn about his/her ways of coping. While not all children display scars and symptoms of sexual abuse, all adult survivors begin to exhibit symptoms at some time during exploration and healing. Watch for the signs and help your partner heal. The following exercise may help you learn more about your partner.

Exercise #3: "Physical, behavioral, emotional, and psychological symptoms that I see in my partner."

Take out a sheet of paper and a pencil. Now, relax, and close your eyes for a moment. Visualize your partner. Recall the information you've learned so far in this book.

What do you see more clearly now as a result of your reading? What are you able to see that you missed before?

Open your eyes. Make a list of any signs that your partner has been sending—whether physically, behaviorally, emotionally, or psychologically.

Chapter 3
Coping for Survival

How Did and Does the Survivor Cope?

People who survive sexual abuse are affected rapidly and permanently. Even after your partner learns to identify and accept his/her feelings about what happened, an irrevocable scar will remain behind with the memories. Although the impacts of sexual abuse differ between individuals, survivors often find that they have been affected in similar ways and have used common strategies to survive.

While these coping strategies allowed the survivor to manage the abusive situation to the best of his/her ability, these methods may become unnecessary (and ineffective) when the survivor finally escapes from the abusive relationship. Unfortunately, coping skills developed in order to tolerate severe physical or emotional trauma are generally associated with primal instincts to ensure survival, and are often difficult to discard (even when they are no longer of use or benefit). Laura readily identified her hypervigilance as problematic:

> *It's hard, you know, to talk about my mother. I mean, she hurt me pretty bad. Not just then, either; somehow she's still messing me with me now. I can't seem to get out of this habit: whenever I come home, I have to check the shower stall, you know, to see if anyone's in there, waiting for me. That's where Mama used to trap me, you know, because the water would be running and no one could hear me screaming in there. It's been over a long time now, and I know it's crazy, but I just can't seem to stop it. Sometimes, I even check two or three times while I'm home, just to make sure.*

Additionally, your partner may discover that the very coping strategies that helped him/her survive the sexual abuse impede your sexual relationship. These effects are discussed further in Chapter 4.

Individuals who have endured sexual abuse, whether as children or adolescents, used psychological and behavioral coping strategies to endure the abuse. These methods, and other coping strategies developed over time, are used by survivors to manage their memories.

Psychological Coping Strategies

Some psychological coping strategies used by a child or an adolescent include denial, humor, an internal locus of control, minimization, rationalization, selective memory, mind/body splitting and spacing out, psychic numbing, psychological disintegration or dissociation, and mental illness.

Denial is a primitive, though fairly common, coping strategy used by individuals experiencing various conflicts or traumas. Denial, or failing to acknowledge that certain events have taken place, is a "stalling" technique. When an individual is unable to withstand the shock of a traumatic event, he/she may mentally "stall" in order to adapt to the new conditions. When he/she is better able to manage, denial is replaced by other, more adaptive coping strategies. While it may be hard for you to believe that your partner could simply deny that the abuse occurred, this may have been the only coping option available to him/her, especially if he/she was very young. While denial is frequently observed among children and adolescents who have been physically and/or sexually abused, it is also employed frequently during the grief process. (If your significant other died, did you ever say to yourself, "This isn't happening! This can't be happening!"? Or have you ever "forgotten" that the person was dead, during the first few months after his/her death?)

Humor can provide emotional distance from others, as well as elevate one's mood. While some survivors use sarcasm and cynical remarks to fulfill their aggressive urges toward their perpetrators, others take shelter in the warmth of lighter humor and laughter. These folks believe that if they continue to laugh, they can keep their tears at bay!

Both denial and humor, as well as most other coping strategies, help the survivor to retain some amount of psychological control over the abusive situation. It is commonly believed that a sense of control over one's environment is primary to the development and maintenance of an individual's personal identity. In a situation in which the individual is unable to physically command his/her environment, he/she may turn to coping methods which facilitate emotional or psychological control over the situation.

To use such coping concepts, the individual must first assume an *internal locus of control*. While many of us inherently maintain an internal locus of control, others believe that their lives and environments are controlled by external forces that are beyond their control. In the abusive situation, the victim may try to concentrate on thoughts, feelings, images, and sensations that he/she can control, in order to avoid those over which he/she has no control. An "externally oriented" person may shift to an internal locus of control to cope with trauma.

During her rape by her stepbrother, who physically outweighed her by more than one hundred pounds, Beth realized she would be unable to escape his grasp. As he began to tear at her nightclothes, she focused on rolling the two of them off her bed and onto the floor, so that she could "protect" the safety and comfort of her bed from the obscenity of his sexual violence. Although Beth was unable to escape the rape, she was able to use her internal locus of control to determine at least one aspect of the situation, enabling her to avoid some of the intense feelings of helplessness that may have otherwise emotionally disabled her.

While Beth used physical force to gain some psychological control, other survivors have relied on mental strategies to achieve the same goal. Some of the psychological forms of coping include minimization, selective memory, and rationalization.

Minimization enables the survivor to believe that his/her abuse was relatively harmless when compared to traumas that others have experienced. *Selective memory* makes it possible for the survivor to recall only non-threatening events, similar to the action of denial. While minimizing the abuse and/or forgetting the events may protect the survivor from the emotional intensity of his/her experiences, it is likely that the survivor will be unable to fully recover from the sexual abuse until the trauma is fully recognized.

Rationalization resembles minimization and selective memory as it, too, mentally empowers the survivor. Instead of blocking or changing the reality of the abuse, the process of rationalization allows a survivor to lend reason to the situation through the invention of excuses for the perpetrator and his/her behavior. Lindsay relates a common rationale for her abuse:

*My father worked very hard when I was small.
There were ten of us, and no matter how hard he
worked, the money never seem to go far enough.
My mother tried to take care of us, but I think it
was too much or her. She used to have to nap in
the afternoon, while we did our chores, and I think
she drank her way through most days. She just
wasn't ever capable of meeting my father's needs
after dealing with us all day. My father was a good
man underneath it all, but I don't think my mother
even made herself available to him. My father
needed to love and desire, and to be loved and
desired, and since I was the oldest, it became my
responsibility when she could no longer do that
for him.*

When the sexual abuse is more severe, or when other coping
mechanisms fail, survivors may turn to some psychological
coping strategies that facilitate a mind/body split. There are
several degrees of splitting, ranging from spacing out to
dissociation.

Spacing out allows the individual to take a break from the
current situation. For whatever reason, the individual
consciously or unconsciously decides that a particular situation,
experience, or feeling is intolerable, and uses his/her mental
powers to remove him/herself. Most of us can recall sitting in
classes which didn't hold our interest, and floating off into
daydreams which were more satisfying than the class.

While most of us daydream when we are excited or bored,
spacing out or splitting generally occurs when a person feels
that his/her life or sense of self is in danger, and that he/she is
unable to escape the impending events. Spacing out permits
the helpless victim to mentally take control of the unbearable
situation, by allowing him/her to flee to a more pleasant and
harmless state. LeVon describes how she learned to split:

*I remember him lifting me up and pressing my
body to his, as he cooed and spoke those crude
words to me. He rapidly became excited and began
to fondle me, and I knew that if I played my cards*

right, that's all I'd have to endure. I gagged with repulsion, disgust and fear, as I stared out the window behind us. Funny how I've never forgotten the details of that window! I learned to play both parts of the game pretty quickly, to let him have what he wanted so he wouldn't hurt me, and to mentally escape through that window so that he couldn't hurt me. It takes years for most pilots to earn their wings, but I learned to fly when I was six years old...

While LeVon escaped the physical and emotional pain by spacing out to a more serene environment outside, other survivors describe a more prominent mind/body split.

In his book, *The Future of Immortality*, R. J. Lifton uses the term, "psychic numbing" to describe one of the psychological coping patterns used by survivors of the nuclear detonation at Hiroshima. He suggested that many of these survivors psychologically generated a desensitization, or numbing, in order to avoid the emotional impact of the horrifying mental images and memories with which they were left.

Similarly, many female survivors recall numbing parts of their bodies so that they would not experience pain in those parts that were being sexually violated. A number of these women also recalled splitting completely out of their bodies, and observing the abuse from above or outside. This more extreme form of *dissociation* and depersonalization was described by Blanca when asked how she had survived the rape by her brother-in-law:

Evan and I were pretty good friends, you know, 'cause of Mira, so I didn't really think much of it when he asked me to meet him at the apartment. When Mira didn't show up like he said she would, we settled down on the couch to wait. Well, I'd had a long day at work, and when he offered me a joint, I said, 'Yeah, OK.' I took a couple of hits (which was stupid 'cause it must've numbed my brain or something, otherwise I would have seen what was coming), but then he starts climbing all over me, and I'm yelling, 'Hey, what the hell are you doing?' But he didn't care what I was yelling. Evan's a pretty big guy, and even though I tried to push him away, he was too heavy. And even though I knew something bad was happening to me, all I could think of was Mira. What if Mira came home while he was on top of me? She would never be able to forgive me! And as I started to think about how horrible that would be, I noticed that I was no longer on the couch. It was then that I saw us below me: Evan pounding away at me, his elbow in my mouth so I couldn't scream anymore, and my eyes focused on the front door. I couldn't believe that Evan was fucking that woman down there, right when Mira was supposed to come home! And I didn't realize that she was me, or that sex was rape, until much later, when I was alone, and safe, and the memories flooded back.

As Blanca points out, dissociation can result in some memory loss. The memory failure, like the dissociation itself, is designed to facilitate survival. While the abuse victim may be unable to emotionally withstand the violence being committed against him/her at the time of the event and may need the psychological respite of dissociation, memories and emotions associated with the abuse often return when the survivor is finally able to tolerate their impacts. For a description of the *depersonalization* process, see the following Informational Highlight.

Informational Highlight
Depersonalization

How many times have you heard stories told by people who endured near-death experiences, asserting that they had floated above their bodies and watched the events below? These people, like many abuse survivors, undergo a process of depersonalization, or mind/body split, which allows them to distance from the crisis at hand. In this way, they are able to experience it as witnesses rather than as participants.

When reporting dreams and memories, many abuse survivors describe the process as "watching home movies" or "viewing videos" as they recall and "see" themselves being violated (experiencing the trauma from an eagle's eye view rather than through their own eyes (first person perspective).

When splitting and spacing out tactics are unsuccessful, survivors may experience more extreme psychological disintegration, and develop a *mental illness*. Research suggests that about twenty percent of survivors experience serious psychological distress during adulthood.[7] While it is difficult to prove that psychological trauma causes mental illness, it does appear that mental illnesses such as Post-traumatic Stress Disorder, Borderline Personality Disorder, Major Depressive Disorder, Obsessive Compulsive Disorder, and Multiple Personality Disorder are frequently associated with early (and often severe) trauma.

Not all survivors develop mental illnesses or personality disorders, but many do experience some recurrent debilitating symptoms. If you are unsure of how your partner has been affected, or would like further information about any of the psychological disorders, look at the Informational Highlights in the next few pages.

Informational Highlight
Post-traumatic Stress Disorder

While Post-traumatic Stress Disorder, or PTSD, is generally thought to be an effect of physical, emotional, or sexual abuse, it might also be described as a coping strategy. Just as other mental disorders allow the survivor to cope with the disturbing reality of his/her life, PTSD "contains" those experiences through various symptoms and behaviors.

If your partner has PTSD, he/she may be experiencing some or all of the following symptoms:

- frequent "reexperiences" of the trauma through recurrent negative images, memories, nightmares, or thoughts
- dread or fear that the event will happen again
- distress or helplessness when exposed to "reminders" of the trauma
- avoidance of those reminders or of people, places, and sensations associated with the trauma
  (In more severe cases, survivors may actually "forget" what has happened and may totally shut down their feelings as well.)
- hopelessness about the past, present and future
- decreased or increased physical/mental activity
- survivors may suffer from:
  - insomnia
  - constant agitation
  - angry outbursts
  - impaired concentration
  - hypervigilance
  - increased sensitivity (includes an extreme startle response)

While not all survivors experience recovery in the same way, many fit the description set forth for PTSD. Most survivors can recall countless times when they have flashed on images of their abuse, and reexperienced the trauma of the past. Others have no memory of their abuse, or recall only terrifying fragments. Many survivors find it incredibly painful to be reminded of thoughts, feelings, actions and situations from their childhood, and frequently opt for a restricted emotional and psychological existence.

Amidst the subdued voices of the past, there is rage, fear, and pain that somehow finds a voice in frequent bouts of irritability, nervous energy, limited concentration, and hypervigilance. And, while some survivors find this repressed life satisfying enough, there are a great number who seek professional assistance because they can no longer endure the lifeless life.

Another mental disorder which shares some of the symptoms of PTSD is Borderline Personality Disorder. While there have been numerous actors of stage and screen who have played roles fraught with Borderline characteristics, in 1987, Glenn Close put the Borderline Personality on the media map, with her portrayal of the excessively willful Alex in Fatal Attraction. Close's portrayal of Alex presented the world with the classic "Borderline," whose symptoms and characteristics included hostile dependency and dangerous manipulation. For a more detailed description, see the Informational Highlight on Borderline Personality Disorder.

Informational Highlight
Borderline Personality Disorder

If your partner has the following symptoms, he/she may suffer from Borderline Personality Disorder:

- intense, chaotic intimate relationships
- reckless behavior
- unpredictable anger
- frequent temper tantrums
- irritability or intense mood swings
- thoughts about or attempts to suicide
- desperate fear of rejection and abandonment
- negative self-image and low self-esteem
- chronic feelings of emptiness and boredom

Individuals with Borderline Personality Disorder view the world with an "all or nothing" perspective. Partners and support providers either love or hate them, according to the "Borderline." Individuals who cope with their worlds in this way, either rule the world or completely submit to its processes. Everything is wonderful and organized, or everything is dirty, bad and chaotic.

This kind of splitting is often the earmark of severe physical and sexual abuse in childhood, where parents and other authority figures either cared for them, or hurt them terribly, where even "good little girls" could not escape submission to Daddy or Mommy's wrath or intrusion, nor the subsequent perceptions of their own "badness." The Borderline Personality develops as the small child learns to cope with the ambivalent chaos around him/her in the only way possible.

A third mental illness which is fairly common to survivors (and which may accompany PTSD) is Major Depressive Syndrome, or what some call Clinical Depression. For a more in-depth look at Depression, see the Informational Highlight.

Informational Highlight

Clinical Depression

Many couples, coping with sexual abuse issues, may become depressed at some point. You may recognize the following symptoms in yourself or in your partner:

- lack of appetite
- under- or overeating
- rapid weight loss or gain
- insomnia or hypersomnia (increased desire to sleep)
- withdrawal from friends and family
- lack of interest or pleasure in activities
- tearfulness
- feelings of hopelessness
- suicidal feelings

People may become depressed for many reasons. Some of the factors which promote depression include:

- biochemical or hormonal imbalance
- poor diet
- lack of exercise
- insufficient social, emotional, or intellectual stimulation
- emotionally hurtful or abusive family life
- limited support system
- substance abuse and chemical dependency
- violence against self or others

Many people wonder what purpose depression serves. Some believe that depression is the physical manifestation of chemical imbalance. Others suggest that depression is rage felt toward others but deflected inward, in order to avoid annihilation of those at whom the rage was initially targeted. Depression may be most simply described as: the process which occurs when one experiences emotions that are too overwhelming, and adaptive coping strategies are not available: one presses the experience down to a more tolerable level.

The energy consumed by this process comes from other sources, and this results in energy reductions such as decreased capacity for attention and/or concentration ("I can't believe I've read this page four times already, and I still don't remember what I've read!), diminished appetite, increased fatigue, psychomotor retardation ("He looks so sluggish today! He's hardly moved from his easy chair."), increased desire for sleep, diminished interest or pleasure ("This has always cheered me up in the past, but it just doesn't seem to be doing the trick today"), and depressed mood.

In light of the incredible obstacles for survival posed by sexual abuse, depression appears to be a natural response to the trauma. Given the quieting aspect of depression, the survivor can "collect" his/her resources without notice by others. It is possible that depression may even be the first step in recovery, as the survivor carefully puts the pieces of his/her life back together, without risking further vulnerability to the perpetrator (e.g. further abuse).

Another fairly common psychiatric disorder which may accompany abuse or trauma is Obsessive Compulsive Disorder. Some of the symptoms of Obsessive Compulsive Disorder are reviewed in the Informational Highlight.

Informational Highlight

Obsessive Compulsive Disorder

If you have been wondering if those little "quirks" or "rituals" that you or your partner perform are unhealthy, you may want to scan the following symptoms of OCD:

- Obsessions are recurrent, persistent thoughts or ideas which the individual experiences as intrusive and out-of-control
- Compulsions are repetitive behaviors or activities which are performed in response to obsessions or obsessive rules
- Compulsions and obsessions are difficult to stop, even when the person tries
- Obsessions and compulsions require a good deal of time and energy of the individual
- Obsessions and compulsions interfere with the daily routine and prevent positive spontaneity
- Obsessions and compulsions are perceived as excessive and unreasonable

One of the most common complaints of survivors is that they have some compulsive behavior over which they feel they have little control. Diane describes her compulsion below:

> *I come home from work and I'm tired, and even though Robert is there, all I can really see is the dirt, and I have to clean. It particularly bothers me when the bathroom is dirty, because, well, it's just not right. I know that the house can't really be accumulating that much dirt while I'm at work, but I just have to get rid of it, especially when Robert is there. I feel like I can't breathe if he and the dirt are there.*

Sometimes, the compulsion to clean reflects the survivor's impaired self-image. If a survivor sees herself as damaged or dirty, because of the abuse, she may try to reduce her anxiety about the feelings by controlling dirt in a material form (e.g. on the floor or shelves). If she can clean the dirt from the floor, she may feel cleaner herself.

The last mental illness to be mentioned here is Multiple Personality Disorder.* It is considered by some to be a severe form of Post-traumatic Stress Disorder. This *psychological integration failure* was described for the public at large in F. R. Schreiber's ground-breaking book and movie, "Sybil." While some practitioners are unsure whether MPD really exists, there are many clinicians who have worked countless hours with patients suffering from the symptoms comprising this disorder. For further description of Multiple Personality Disorder, see the Informational Highlight.

The majority of those who suffer from MPD have been traumatized or abused as youngsters. One research group even claimed that, during one of their research projects, they discovered that nearly 83% of the subjects diagnosed with MPD had experienced childhood sexual abuse, and that 68% of that group had survived incest.[8] The research suggests that many abuse survivors begin to split off their personalities as early as age five.

---

* (Now labelled *Dissociative Identity Disorder* by the psychology profession.)

Informational Highlight

Multiple Personality Disorder

Individuals with MPD generally have two or more distinct personalities which alternately control their physical form and other personality "fragments." These "alter egos" usually differ significantly from one another (even in gender, ethnic background, and sexual preference), and as a personality "comes up" to take control, the individual's speech, facial expression, comportment, posture, handedness, and manner may change. If the individual, or the first alternate personality is unable to control or manage the individual's painful feelings, a new alternate personality or fragment will be split off and developed to meet those needs.

While it's hard to assess the extent and pervasive nature of this mental illness, Linda Walker, whose clinical practice in California consists solely of clients with MPD, suggests that she has treated clients with as many as 384 personalities and "fragments" (that's 384 in a single client!). While this number of fragmentations seems extraordinary, it is also quite likely that an even greater number of fragments go undetected, even to the most highly-trained clinician.

Some of the symptoms of multiplicity include:

- limited concentration
- confusion
- severe headaches
- fear
- panic
- self-destructive behavior
- intense irritability or mood swings
- time loss
- "forgotten" or unexpected travel
- "forgotten" or unexpected purchases
- behavior reported by others which is considered inconsistent with "normal" routine/self-image

As alternate personalities fade to the background, and the dominant or original personality comes forth, the individual may be confused about her/his actions, thoughts, feelings, or experiences. She/he may not recall the feelings and experiences of the alternate personality. Due to these bouts of amnesia, she/he may have to become adept at lying to or distracting those who inquire about her/his previous whereabouts and/or actions.

Dissociation, or mentally fleeing the traumatic situation, may have been the only way for some to survive. An even fewer number of survivors had to actually split-off the part of themselves that was being abused in order to survive. And to those individuals, their "alternate selves" were psychic saviors.

The majority of sexual abuse survivors used less extreme coping strategies to manage their traumas. Many of the psychological coping strategies that may have been utilized have already been discussed, but survivors likely also employed some behavioral coping methods.

Behavioral Coping Strategies

Some of the common behavioral coping strategies used by survivors include active and passive response, addiction (to chemicals, food, gambling), the maintenance of absolute control over other aspects of daily life, somatization, and forms of biofeedback.

Many survivors were sexually abused as children while they were sleeping or in bed. While it may be difficult for you to accept, your partner may have chosen to respond passively by pretending that he/she was asleep. In this way, your partner may have been able to feel that he/she had not allowed the abuser the satisfaction of wakeful submission. Your partner may even remember thinking, "He may be able to abuse me, but I don't have to let him know that I feel or hear him."

Other survivors may have chosen to respond more actively. These individuals acknowledged their physical stimulation and allowed their bodies to respond with pleasure to avoid the physical tension or pain of abuse. These survivors may also have taken a more active role in the abuse, and may even have sought out sexual interactions with their abusers after the initial abuse.

It may be difficult for you to understand that even though your partner may have chosen to use an active response to manage the trauma, the sexual interactions are still defined as abuse. The active form of responding, like all other coping strategies, allowed the survivor to experience a sense of control over atrocities committed against him/her, which reduced some of the overwhelming feelings of helplessness caused by the abuse. If the survivor's world was devoid of other attention, he/she may have sought further contact with the perpetrator following the onset of abuse. Many survivors recall feeling that "something was better than nothing."

Unfortunately, due to the active nature of this coping strategy, many survivors begin to doubt themselves after responding in this way, and may come to believe that they were responsible for the abuse. They were not. No one *deserves* to have their dignity, self-respect, and sense of self, stripped from them by another human being.

Another form of control used by survivors is the absolute regulation of other aspects of daily life. This may be reflected as a magnified interest (e.g. the sexually abused child who excels in school, the arts, or sports), a tightly organized schedule, or even as a compulsion. The idea is for the survivor to experience so much control over the other aspects of his/her life that the powerlessness of the abuse is less debilitating than it might otherwise be.

There are two other behavioral coping mechanisms which employ the concept of control: biofeedback and somatization. Biofeedback, or use of physical sensations and mental processes to control the body, may have been employed by your partner to "control the damage": during or after the abuse, the survivor can psychically numb or anesthetize parts of his/her body that are being or have been abused, in order to avoid the experience of pain (whether it is physical or mental). Survivors may also choose to inflict pain on their own limbs or digits, in order to experience greater control over their pain. Melanie describes some of her coping methods below:

> *I remember that I used to stare at my ceiling when my step-brother abused me. I always wished I could just become part of the paint on that ceiling, just fade right into it. Sometimes, that just wasn't enough; and when it hurt so bad that I didn't think I would make it, I would just bite the inside of my cheek until I could taste blood. It hurt, but at least the hurt was mine. For those few moments in time, Steve wasn't hurting me, I was.*

Another way that survivors may have used their bodies (and may continue to use their bodies) to manage their feelings about the sexual abuse is through somatization. Somatization is the belief and experience of illness, even when organic pathology is absent. Survivors who somatically react may experience a variety of gastro-intestinal, cardiopulmonary, pseudo-neurologic, sexual and pain symptoms, when they repress their painful or "unacceptable" feelings.

Use of the body in this way may be one of the only ways that a child survivor can express his/her feelings about the sexual abuse, as he/she may be unable to discuss the abuse, or associated feelings, with members of his/her family or support network. LeVon, whose splitting behavior was described earlier in this chapter, complained to her parents of stomach upset and nausea:

> *I'd been working on the abuse issues for a while when I got to the college dorm. Nothing is sacred in the dorm and those girls talked about everything from tampons to bowel movements. And, swear to God, that was the first time I realized that everyone else didn't have diarrhea and nausea all of the time! It sounds disgusting, but until then, I just thought that was normal. I saw a doctor, and he said nothing was wrong with me. Then I started to put it together: after the abuse started, I just always wanted Cray out of me. Every part he'd entered was flushing itself, trying to purify and rid me of that awful man. It took a while, but when I started to forgive my body and took on the responsibility of recognizing how devastated I was that not even my parents recognized that I was "sick," my body started to heal and the physical symptoms started to fade.*

As LeVon noted, sometimes somatization enables the survivor to recognize emotional damage, and other times, somatization is used to identify the extent of the pain to others (e.g. physical complaints might be responded to by the parents, even if they knew nothing of the sexual abuse).

At the other end of the behavioral coping continuum is addiction. While addiction (to chemicals, food, sex, gambling) is not a very healthy coping mechanism, it may allow the survivor to mentally escape the abuse or its haunting memories.

As mentioned previously, abuse and chemical addiction often go hand-in-hand. Just as perpetrators may use substances to escape the pain of their own lives, or the guilt of the abuse they have committed, survivors may use chemicals to withstand repeated violations, or to dull distressing memories of the past.

Survivors may also use food addictively, and in fact, eating disorders are quite common among survivors. In Anorexia nervosa, or intentional self-starvation, it is common for the survivor to starve his/her body as a means to gain control over a chaotic or tyrannized life. In Bulimia nervosa, or the Binge-Purge Syndrome, the survivor may experience a massive sense of loss or emptiness (e.g. loss of his/her ideal family life after incest occurs) which he/she may try to cover or fill with food. Yet, the survivor soon discovers that food is not an adequate bandage, and that the amount consumed in the process is too overwhelming for the system, thus causing regurgitation.

The survivor who suffers from Bulimia may also binge in response to painful or intolerable feelings that arise from the abuse, thus using food to "stuff" the feelings back down, so that they may be swallowed along with the food. Most survivors find that using food in this manner is also ineffective, and quite often, the feelings are more powerful than the food, and force it back up.

Finally, there are those survivors who eat in their "cloak of chaos," or the frenetic activity state some take on when they don't want to recognize the painful reality of their abuse. These survivors generally eat in an out-of-control fashion, then force themselves to purge later, in response to derogatory, judgmental self-statements (e.g. "Look at all that crap you just ate! You're a bad person who can't even control herself/himself!").

Another addiction (which is often thought to be a pleasant activity), is gambling. For the individual who survives through the cloak of chaos, and seeks out excitement to avoid recognizing internal trauma, gambling may serve to quiet or contain the violated self. As with the other addictions, gambling may offer the survivor a semblance of control over his/her life, though this control is likely tenuous and fleeting.

Even though survivors may use a variety of psychological and behavioral coping skills, these may be inadequate to manage the intense feelings and memories associated with their abuse. As a result, survivors may become suicidal at some points in their lives.

Relatively few survivors actually complete suicide when compared to those who contemplate or attempt suicide. Suicide threats cannot be taken lightly. For more information about dealing with suicidal feelings in your partner, see the Informational Highlight.

Informational Highlight
Suicide and crisis management

If you were to survey your community, it's likely that you would find that most people have thought about suicide at some point in their lives. Generally, those thoughts develop when folks feel down, depressed, and hopeless about the future. Frequently, the passage of time is sufficient to fade away these lethal thoughts and people move on. For some, the option of suicide becomes more prominent over time rather than less so.

If you are worried that your partner may be suicidal, look for the following signs:

- hopelessness (can't seem to visualize anything in the future)
- focus on the past, especially on negative or traumatic events
- withdrawing from friends and family
- saying good-bye to friends and family
- "tying up loose ends"
- giving away favorite items
- openly talking about suicide and death
- change in behavior (after a period of depression, your partner suddenly becomes more active)
- acquiring the means to kill self
- writing suicide notes

If your partner is experiencing any combination of these symptoms, speak to him/her openly and honestly about your suspicions. Do not hesitate to ask the survivor if he/she is considering suicide. If your partner is suicidal, seek help immediately. Most hospitals and clinics have 24-hour hotlines that you can call for assistance. If your partner is actively attempting suicide, dial 911 and ask for immediate assistance. Whatever course you take, be sure that you and your partner get the help that you need.

Coping strategies, no matter how adaptive or healthy they may appear, can only facilitate management of feelings, situations and memories associated with sexual abuse. Sexual abuse can not be erased, and it stays with the survivor forever, no matter how many years pass between the abuse and recovery. All survivors bear scars, though some are more visible than others. Now that you are involved in this process, you may bear your own scars.

Exercise #4: "Coping skills that my partner and I use"

Sit quietly for five minutes and visualize your partner.

What are the coping skills that he/she uses each day?
Do these change when things get really tough?

Now study yourself for a few minutes.

What are the strategies that you use to cope?
Do these change when things get really tough?

Chapter 4
Impacts on Sexuality

- What is the difference between sexuality and sensuality?
- How can sexuality and sensuality be affected by sexual abuse?
- Can sexuality and sensuality be healed?
- How does the partner fit in?

Even though womankind has developed more fully since the dawn of the sexual revolution, sexuality continues to be a troublesome enigma to many women. In an age in which women fight for status and equality in the work place, they are often resistant to expressing their sensuality and sexuality, for fear that they will not be taken seriously, or that they will be harassed by their male co-workers. Unfortunately, this suppression of sexuality and sensuality forces the individual to omit part of her sense of self, and part of her knowledge, experience and understanding of the world.

Sensuality vs. Sexuality

Sensuality generally refers to those qualities which suggest to self and others that one gains pleasure from being man or woman. Your partner may choose a particular style of clothing to express his/her sensuality because of the way that the fabric feels and fits against the body, in a fashion which emphasizes the masculine or feminine form.

Another way that men and women express their sensuality is in their hair. Native-American cultures, teach members to take pride in their hair, to care for it well, and to protect its inherent power. Women, who have the power to reproduce, must especially take care of their hair. Other cultures, such as the Muslims, punish women if they uncover their hair for anyone but their husbands, as to do so would be to blatantly flaunt their sensuality. And for survivors, the hair can be an all-too-accessible extension of their sensuality. Sandy comments as follows:

> *After the rape I just wanted to be someone else. I changed everything: my hair, my clothes, my makeup, even my diet and my routine. I lost*

weight, and with my new short cut, I suppose I looked like a boy (safe from other rapists lurking about!). That wore off after a while, and I grew my hair out some, and even allowed myself to wear more feminine styles. Even though I can do those outward things now, nothing's really changed on the inside yet. I was working on a painting the other day and my partner came by and just lightly tousled my hair. Without a thought I jerked my head away and glared at her. It was just Joyce, but for that instant, I was back there, my sexuality being yanked out and spread open for all to see. It was that bastard saying, "Your ass is mine. I'll touch you wherever I please."

Sandy, like many survivors is reactive to others touching her hair. While a survivor may find it pleasant and sensual to have his/her hair stroked while cuddling or making love with his/her partner, the survivor may respond with hostility to uninvited hair tousling.

Somewhat different from sensuality, sexuality is defined as the individual's choice to identify with one sex or the other, and the characteristics associated with that particular gender. In their book Incest and Sexuality, Maltz and Holman suggest that:

"Sexuality refers to how people feel about their bodies and genitals, how they choose to express sexual energy, and how and with whom they prefer to share sexual feelings. In sexual expression, a woman projects her intimate self outward.. On a physical level, individuals can experience pleasurable sensations and tension release, which then reinforce good feelings about the body. On a social level, healthy sexual expression involves intimacy and an exchange of feelings of positive regard and acceptance."[9]

According to some, survivors are especially prone to confuse sexuality with sexual abuse, even though they are intellectually aware of differences between the two. In terms of the definition above, survivors respond to their sexuality quite differently than non-survivors.

Impacts on Sensuality and Sexuality

While you may have learned to accept your body and feel positive about your genitals, your partner is more likely to withdraw from his/her body, even to the point of pretending that his/her body is separate from the rest of him/her.

In numerous sessions, one survivor disclosed that she pretended that she and her body were two separate people. She remarked how odd it felt to be walking along, without feeling for anything below her neck, sensing that she was almost floating in the direction that she needed to go. Like this one, many survivors reject their bodies because they feel that their bodies have betrayed them for responding during the abuse.

Your partner may further encapsulate his/her sexuality by expressing his/her sexual energy in a more extreme fashion than you do. The most common expressions are complete withdrawal of sexual energy, or complete investment in sexualized behavior. Sexual abuse may even sway the survivor's sexual sense of self, leading the survivor to select different kinds of sexual partners and expressions than he/she otherwise might.

Now that you have a better idea of what sensuality and sexuality are, and how these might be interpreted or translated differently for your partner, let's take a more comprehensive look at the impact that sexual abuse has on your partner's sexuality.

If your partner lived in an incestuous home, he/she may not have been exposed to many healthy models of sexuality and affection. While many incest survivors do learn about positive sensuality and sexuality from others in their support networks, such as teachers, friends, and extended family members, the intricate web of secrecy and deception that surrounds incest can stunt self-knowledge. Even if the survivor is able to learn about positive sexuality, he/she may be unable to integrate this knowledge into his/her social reality.

It is believed that survivors who have observed healthy models of sexuality prior to their abuse are more likely to develop a healthy sexuality than those who have not. In non-incestuous families, where abuse occurred outside the home, the survivor's chances of receiving positive messages about his/her body and about sexuality (in general) are greater. Just because a family is not incestuous does not mean that they will naturally promote a healthy sexuality. For instance, very religious families often promote an extremely conservative and chaste model of sexuality for their children, especially their daughters. Sexuality must be cultivated and developed as an individual matures and gains knowledge.

Incest, like most other forms of sexual abuse, leaves the survivor with a very damaged sense of sexual and sensual self. If your partner was asserting his/her sensuality at the time when he/she was abused (e.g. the four-year old girl who parades around the house in her mother's negligee, proclaiming that she will be daddy's wife now, or the ten-year old boy who sends his divorced mother's suitors away from the door, claiming that he is the only man that she needs), your partner may feel that these assertions have been punished, and he/she may be unlikely to assert sensuality in the same manner. Helena, who was molested by her father at age ten, recalls how the incest began and the effects that it has had on her sensuality:

> I remember how I used to sit in front of my bureau to brush my hair at night. 'One hundred strokes to perfection,' my mother used to tell me. So I would sit and brush and brush until my dark hair shone. I recall seeing commercials, where the actress was seated in front of the mirror in a white negligee, brushing her hair. She always looked so happy, I thought. But when my father began to come into my room to watch me brush my hair at night, I didn't feel very happy. At first, he just sat on my bed and watched me, but after a couple of times, he began to stand next to me. Then finally one night, he closed the door to my room, and he sat right behind me, with his chest pressed against my back, and he told me how much he liked to watch me brush my hair. As I began to brush, he lifted his hands to my tiny breasts and began to stroke me. I loved my daddy, and I didn't want to make him angry, but I wanted him to stop, but he wouldn't, not even when I asked him to. He let one hand drop to my vagina, and commanded me to keep brushing while he continued to fondle me. He didn't stop until he came, then he left my room

quickly without another word. He abused me several more times before I finally told my teacher, and then he denied to her what he'd done. He never came into my room after that, but he never apologized either. I wear my hair very short now, because I just can't bear to brush it; it just makes me feel too damn vulnerable. But I don't like to do many things about my appearance; I'd rather just do my job and go by unnoticed.

Even if your partner was not asserting his/her sensuality at the time of the abuse, it is still likely that damage was incurred to his/her sensuality and sexuality. Often survivors do not take an interest in their appearance; they may add or lose weight to make themselves less physically attractive or to hide their sexuality.

Survivors may also achieve this by wearing loose or androgynous clothing. Female survivors may even adapt their speech and mannerisms to less closely resemble that of women, in order to deter interactions with men.

Many survivors experience numerous changes in sexuality after being abused and after beginning a healing process. After an individual is sexually abused, he/she may feel betrayed by his/her body—especially if it functioned accurately and responded to the sexual stimulation. Similar to other organs, an individual's genitals are designed to receive sensory information and react accordingly. In response to sexual stimulation, the body will increase blood flow to the genitals, making them more sensitive to any kind of touch.

Sensations in a woman's genitals may cause lubrication in the vagina, facilitating intercourse and increasing the capacity for pleasure. Sensations in the male's genitals cause the penis to become erect so that intercourse can be possible. While it is difficult for most survivors to recognize the responses that their bodies may have made to the abusive sexual stimulation, the healing process requires that the survivor learns to forgive his/her body for its "hard wiring."

In addition to general feelings of resentment toward his/her body, your partner may encounter various other problems and conflicts with sexuality. Some of those issues identified by survivors include:

- problems with sexual desire and pleasure
  (including fear of the unknown sexual entity,
  healthy sexuality and sexual pleasure)
- compulsive sexual activity or inactivity
- a need for total control during sex (to avoid
  sexual and emotional vulnerability)
- keeping "tuned in" during sex
- sexual exploitation
- the use of sex to fulfill emotional needs
- flashbacks during sex

Sometimes, these symptoms develop in specific combinations which affect one's feelings and beliefs about sexuality. Some of the more common patterns for survivor sexuality include:

- refusal of sexuality
- emphasis on blatant sexuality
- need for total control during sex
- emphasis on fears associated with the
  original abuse

When a survivor refuses to integrate his/her sexuality, a number of behaviors, thoughts and feelings become intolerable and unacceptable. The survivor strives to exist as an entity without sexuality. Sexual thoughts, even those as non threatening as lighthearted fantasy, are deemed "bad," and repressed so that they will not impinge on the survivor's sense of security.

Sexual behaviors and feelings, including sexual desire and sexual pleasure, are similarly avoided. When the survivor feels that he/she must engage in sexual behavior, he/she may call in some "psychological reinforcements" or coping skills (such as dissociation), so that he/she can space out during "unacceptable actions" (such as sexual touching and intercourse). While numbing or "leaving" the body allows the survivor to avoid feelings associated with his/her sexuality, it can become problematic for the survivor who wants to develop healthy sexual functioning. Dissociation prohibits the experience of any real pleasure or joy generated during sexual interaction. As dissociation becomes more automatic, it increasingly inhibits the experience of sexual pleasure. Yvonne describes the "non-sexual self" that she began to develop after being sexually abused by a neighbor:

> I don't remember the first couple of years after it happened, but by sixth grade, I had developed this 'persona'. I wanted to have fun, but I couldn't really enjoy things the way that other children could. I wanted to learn, but academics weren't enough. I wanted to be a cheerleader, but simply couldn't stand to be noticed that much. I finally gave up one day, and tried to kill myself. I was ten years old, and I wanted to die. I botched the job; now I can say, 'Thank God!' After that, I figured that since I hadn't died, God must be watching out for me. So I worked toward piousness and I tried to become a nun. That made my life easy, because then I didn't have to deal with the sexual abuse, or with boys, or with a social life, or with the disgust I felt when I heard other people talking about sex. When I fell in love the first time was when I realized that there had to be another way to deal with the stuff that happened to me.

Yvonne demonstrates how well the rejection of her sexuality served her needs... for a while. Then, when she recognized that she desired some part of her sexual self, it became necessary to manage her feelings about the sexual abuse in a different manner.

Some survivors vow to never integrate their sexuality, and they may remain separate, isolated and "safe" from intimate interactions. They may become androgynous or "sexually neutral" and choose to wear short hair and loose, non-descript clothing.

Female survivors may work or play at activities which are not typically feminine. They may become "tomboys," which further decreases the risk of experiencing vulnerability associated with being female. Not all survivors who fail to integrate sexuality choose to be tomboys. Some continue to value their femininity after the abuse, but they work hard to prohibit anyone else from perceiving them as attractive or "available." These survivors may safeguard their bodies and spirits by becoming extremely religious, claiming celibacy as the only moral choice. Some actually enter convents or seminaries to avoid further sexual contact.

Other survivors emphasize blatant sexuality, at the expense of other facets of their personalities. A stereotypical example might be found in the prostitute who was abused as a child, and because of his/her feelings of worthlessness and hopelessness, integrates only sexuality and fails to develop his/her intellectual, emotional or spiritual self. These survivors have generally experienced a massive blow to their self-esteem as a result of sexual abuse—perceiving themselves to be devoid of anything of value except their sexuality. Several studies suggest that as many as eighty percent of prostitutes are survivors of child or adolescent sexual abuse, who ran away to escape a perpetrator and turned to prostitution as a means of financial survival.

Survivors who over-incorporate sexuality in this way may also exploit sexuality. While the stereotype of the prostitute is a little extreme, use of sexuality to manage psychological issues is more common than you may realize. Some survivors, such as the prostitute in the example above, may flaunt their sexuality because they feel that they have little else of value. These survivors become sexual doormats for others to use, exploit and discard. This emphasis on sexuality reflects a passive or submissive stance to the survivor's sexual identity.

Other survivors attempt to use their sexual selves to assert control over others, in response to the archaic feelings of powerlessness. This desire for control may range from the desire to control sexual interactions to the desire to sexually exploit others.

In Chapter 2, Ann described her sexual addiction (and how sex allowed her to manage feelings of worthlessness, emotional chaos, and powerlessness). Her desire to repress and contain these feelings and to control others prompted her to have sex with as many partners as she could find.

Survivors may also use sex as a means to attain nurturing. For this reason, a survivor might seek compulsive sexual activity in an attempt to fill the emotional void experienced as a result of the abuse. It would be unlikely for this survivor to refuse any sexual requests or demands, for fear that he/she would lose the source of emotional sustenance.

Susan recounts part of her story:

I grew up way too fast because of the abuse. I was just a baby when it happened, so by the time I got to high school, I didn't really think twice about my "virginity." So when I met Anthony, I assumed we'd have sex sometime. He was so sweet, and he understood me so well, and he listened to me, and held me. So when he said, "Baby, if you love me, you'll do this," I just figured, "Sure, OK, I want to hang on to this guy. I love how he makes me feel, so pure and clean, and I don't want to lose that." So we did it. And we did it, and we did it. Until he got tired of me, and moved on. Then I had to find a new boyfriend, because I wanted to feel understood and loved like that again. Love. Yeah, right.

Even if the survivor does not seek sexual interaction compulsively, he/she may turn to sex when feeling emotions of any sort. If the abuse occurred in childhood, the survivor may have developed simple associations between sex and emotional distress of any kind. And when later partners have offered support and warmth during sexual interactions, the survivor learns to use sex to manage her/his feelings (as well as avoiding additional unpleasant feelings, such as rejection by a partner).

Finally, your partner's sexuality may reflect his/her fear of the original abuse. While most survivors experienced fear during the abuse, many continue to experience fear even after the abuse has ended. These survivors may want to limit sexuality in order to avoid flashbacks and "reminders." These survivors are likely to experience an incredible aversion to sexual interaction, to lack sexual desire and/or pleasure, may have difficulties becoming sexually aroused, achieving orgasm, staying "tuned in" during sex, and may also experience flashbacks during sex. In other words, every time the survivor tries to interact sexually with a partner, he/she feels as if the abuse were occurring all over again (no matter how sweet and gentle his/her partner may be).

Jill's story reflects her aversion to sex and the flashbacks she experienced:

For the longest time, I didn't try to do anything sexual, and that was just fine with me. By the time I got to college, I started to feel weird and different when my roommates would begin to talk about sex and I'd have nothing to say. They talked a lot about masturbation, "frenching," intercourse, and as disgusted as all that talk made me feel, it felt worse not to "belong." One day, when Anne asked if I wanted to double with her boyfriend and his brother, I agreed to go. The date was OK, as far as dates go, but by the end of the evening, Alan just wouldn't get out of my space. Then, I thought, "well maybe I'll see what all this talk is about," so I tried to relax, but when he rolled on top of me as he was kissing me, I suddenly began to panic and feel nauseous. Voices in my head were screaming, "Get off! Get out! He's going to hurt you!" And I couldn't escape the fear no matter how hard I tried. My abuser's face appeared before my eyes and suddenly I was ten again, helpless and alone. So I shoved him as hard as I could, whimpering, "Stop! Stop!" Until he finally split. I locked the door, and tried to calm down, checking over and over to see if I was OK. After I was sure he wasn't coming back, I set about getting the makeup off my face and discarding the silly clothes that I'd worn on this ill-fated attempt at a "normal" social life.

Most survivors want to have a healthy sexuality and a normal approach to dating. For most, it is an uphill battle. Even those survivors who act blatantly sexual and may appear to know what they're doing, may be hiding behind a sexualized facade to hide confusion they experience about development, social interaction, dating or sexuality.

While you and your partner have been able to develop an intimate relationship, your partner may still have problems with sexual response. Your partner's sexual desire or "libido" may be inhibited or nonexistent, he/she may have difficulty becoming aroused, or may be able to engage in sex, but may be unable to achieve orgasm. Most of these issues reflect the absence of trust by the survivor and a fear of losing control during sexual contact. Ted describes some of his issues below:

> *I really think women are great. I like being around them and I don't think that my abuse has hurt me too much in terms of dating. Well, I don't think so at least. See, I go to clubs, and I watch to see what's what. And, sometimes, I'll be watching these beautiful women and I'll get hornier than hell. I try to control myself when I'm in the club, you know, I don't want to embarrass myself, but when I get that turned on, I gotta meet one of those women. And I'm a pretty good-looking guy, so I do all right. Sometimes, when I leave with a woman, and we're alone, somehow I just can't seem to get fired up.*

At this point, Ted has yet to realize that the restrictions he experiences around sexual arousal may indeed be linked to the sexual abuse that he endured. Many survivors do not attribute their problems to past sexual abuse, especially if they can become aroused or sexually active at times. Alice, on the other hand, was quite capable of seeing the connections between her abuse and her inability to achieve orgasm.

> *I like sex, but I'm not very good at it yet. Somehow, I just can't seem to drop off that cliff at the end, to achieve the final passion, the ultimate. I feel my partner inside me and I am enraptured. I like the ride, and I can even stick with it now, without splitting even once. But when I sense that he is near, and I am ready to explode, this wave of fear comes over me. I feel like if I really let go, something bad will happen, that if I become that vulnerable with him, he will take advantage and hurt me. Then he comes, and I lay back, unsated, disappointed and resentful, jealous, even, that he has gotten what I cannot have.*

In this vignette, clearly, Alice's archaic fears of her abuser and her unwillingness to really trust her partner prohibit her orgasm and sense of sexual fulfillment.

If the abuser was a trusted relative or family friend, your partner may have been frightened by the action of the perpetrator during the abuse. The survivor may have experienced even greater fear that the abuser and others would abandon him/her after the abuse was discovered. In this case, the survivor might have attempted to please the perpetrator to maintain contact and to avoid being hurt further. This attitude may have left him/her unable to say no to sexual demands and requests; or caused him/her to feel vulnerable to sexual exploitation by others.

Given these impacts of sexual abuse, you're probably wondering if your partner can heal the wounds of abuse. For the most part, survivors can learn to integrate the abuse, confront fears, and develop healthy sexuality.

Healing the Sensual and Sexual Self

In order to combat the most generalized effects of sexual abuse, your partner needs to develop positive self-statements and a more positive sense of self. Affirmations can help the survivor to combat negative ideas that he/she developed as a result of abuse. For example, when your partner fails an exam or misses a promotion at work, the negative sense of self that he/she developed early in life may cause him/her to feel like a failure or feel incapable of ever succeeding. He or she may feel shameful and undeserving of success. If your partner has begun to develop self-affirmations, he/she can respond to the "old negative self" with encouragement—such as, "Well, that didn't go well but that doesn't mean I can't succeed next time"; or "I hated not succeeding, so I am going to try harder to get what I want next time."

Your partner may also need to increase his/her ability to nurture the self and to soothe the inner child who remembers the abuse too well. Development of the parenting voice can assist the survivor to experience compassion and empathy for him/herself when things are not going well. When old fears arise, the parenting voice can help soothe and calm the survivor, so that the inner child doesn't exacerbate feelings of fear and helplessness.

To develop a healthy sexuality and sensual self, the survivor may have to seek healthy role models (in colleagues, teachers, doctors, friends, actors or in one's adult children). Your partner will need to take a pain-staking inventory of his/her sexuality to determine what to keep and what to replace with healthier characteristics or ideas. Unless your partner was abused as an infant, there was probably some normal sexual development that occurred prior to the abuse, which will remain as a foundation for the healthy sexual self. This process will increase your partner's awareness of his/her body, socialization, social interaction style, and sexual integration or incorporation.

It is important that you and your partner explore what happened: recognition and integration of all aspects of the abuse can promote healing. If your partner can identify the skeletons in the closet, he/she can pull them out and use the closet for more important functions. Most survivors find it helpful to be able to predict or control some aspects of their responses. Knowing what his/her triggers are can allow your partner to remain in control of his/her life and to actively combat the old fears and demons. Some stimuli which are most often associated with old abuse memories include the following "triggers":

Triggers
- Smells
  - cigarette smoke, alcohol, coffee, onions, sweat, dust, rotting trash, stale air, blood, semen, burning material (clothes, food, flesh)
- Sounds
  - music, arguments, loud voices, tone of voice, particular, spoken words, cursing, "talking dirty," crying babies, laughter, grunting, barking dogs, screaming or whimpering
- Times
  - night, afternoon (e.g. after school), bedtime or nap time, time associated with day care or baby-sitters, seasons, holidays, vacations
- Places
  - "scene of the crime" or places which resemble the site where abuse was endured, unfamiliar places, a baby-sitter's home, darkness, cars, bathrooms, bedrooms, cemeteries, open fields, closets, certain roads, tents, doctor's offices (especially OB/GYN and X-ray departments)
- Events
  - seeing perpetrators or site of abuse, visiting friends associated with time/age of abuse, playing with children whose ages resemble those at which abuse occurred, engaging in similar activities (whether intended as abusive or not), being in certain sexual positions,

dreams, being physically touched or moved by someone, experiencing body memories, being instructed, failing

- Sensations
  - body memories, sexual arousal, sexual responses, touching, feeling dirty, having hair touched, the feel of certain clothing
- Sights
  - children, erotica or pornography, animals, men, certain clothing, gray hair, dirty hair, facial characteristics, large people, dirty, empty or dark houses, rumpled sheets, water
- Interpersonal dynamics
  - personality (manipulative, antisocial, dependent, sociopathic (no remorse, idiosyncratic rules), attitude (self-involved, rigid (all or nothing), low self-esteem), gestures of caring or giving

Exercise #5: "My partner's triggers"

Do you know what your partner's triggers are? Take a few moments and make a list of the things you suspect act as triggers for your partner. When your partner is willing to talk with you about the abuse and its impacts, have him/her review your list. Find out which items you detected correctly and which you left out.

After your partner begins to develop awareness of his/her sensuality and sexuality, it is imperative that he/she begin a healthy exploration of his/her sexuality. Before connecting with you, it is important that your partner learn more about his/her own desires, needs and sexual "hard wiring." Since most survivors associate sexuality with the out-of-control, helpless feelings surrounding the abuse it may benefit the survivor to create new and safer associations for sexuality and sexual interaction.

The exploration process in which your partner can learn about and enjoy his/her body must be private, safe and controlled by your partner. Through this process, the survivor becomes more empowered and confident about his/her sexuality and ability to engage in a mutually-consenting sexual interaction.

Let your partner tell you how you can participate in this sexual healing and how you can be most supportive.

Sexual exploration generally begins with the self-inventory. The inventory is accomplished by the survivor standing in front of a mirror and looking at him/herself. The first time that the exercise is attempted, the survivor may opt to remain clothed. Generally, people feel somewhat uncomfortable staring at themselves in a mirror, so the exercise can be timed in order to decrease some of the anxiety.

Exercise #6: "The self-inventory"

While this exercise is designed for the survivor, you may wish to do a self-inventory as well, in order to get to know your own body. You can choose to do this exercise while clothed or unclothed. Many clients try the exercise the first time while clothed, in order to reduce some of the anxiety. This exercise can be attempted again, unclothed, when doing so is comfortable.

Stand in front of a full-length mirror for about ten minutes. Take note of what you see, and make a mental list of the positives and negatives. After the time has elapsed, write down the pros and cons that you have assessed about your body.

The second time the exercise is attempted, the survivor disrobes in order to begin confronting and processing some negative and positive feelings associated with being nude, being sensual, and being a sexual entity.

Exercise #7: "The nude self-inventory"

When you are comfortable enough to do disrobe and stand in front of a mirror. For the next ten minutes, allow your eyes to scan your face and body.

What do you see?
Which parts do you enjoy about your face and body?
Which parts are more difficult for you to accept?
Are there any parts of your face or body that are positively sensual?

Now, instead of focusing on your body, experience the process of being nude. Allow yourself to experience the way you are holding your body, the way you are standing and the way you look at yourself.

How does it feel to be unclothed?
What do you experience as positive about the exercise?

The exercise can be done as many times and as often as the survivor wishes. The process of disrobing and accepting the way one's body looks and feels may help the survivor accept the body as good and positive.

Exercise #8: "Physical affirmations"

It is important that you and your partner find ways to accept and feel good about your bodies. To promote this process, you can develop affirmations about your bodies. After disrobing, stand in front of a full-length mirror for approximately ten minutes. Determine which parts of your face and body are the features you like most. When you have selected a few to work with, develop positive statements about each of these parts. For instance, if you believe that your eyes are your best feature, you may develop an affirmation such as, "My eyes are beautiful. I like looking at the world through my eyes."

Remember that you can learn to enjoy a variety of things associated with your body, including sight, smell, texture, size, color, taste and function. Be creative with the affirmations you develop for your body. Then use those affirmations whenever you dress or disrobe!

After completing the inventory, it is important that the survivor develop a good working knowledge of his/her genitalia. Many survivors have so distanced themselves from their bodies that they have little idea of how the body functions, nor what all of the components are called! When you and your partner feel comfortable, you may each want to attempt the following exercise.

Exercise #9: "Getting to know your genitalia"

If you are male, you can use a full-length mirror to view your body and genitalia. Spend as much time as you need to observing yourself in the mirror, unclothed.

How many sexual body parts can you name?

Which parts are you having trouble identifying or naming?

If you have difficulty identifying or naming your genitalia, consult a guide for male sexuality in Chapter 10.

If you are female, you will most likely need a hand-mirror (in addition to a full-length mirror) to view all of your sexual body parts. After observing yourself, unclothed in a full-length mirror, see how many sexual body parts you can identify and name.

Which parts do you have trouble identifying or naming?

When you are ready to move on, take your hand mirror and find a comfortable seat on a couch or bed so that you can place the mirror directly under your genitalia. Observe and explore your labia, vulva, clitoris, vagina, and anus. If you have any difficulty identifying these parts, consult a book on female sexuality, such as *For Yourself*. If you wish, you can position yourself to internally explore your vagina, uterus, and ovaries. This internal self-exam is taught at most women's and family planning clinics.

When you and your partner have become more comfortable with visual exploration, you can try tactile exploration—or exploring your bodies with your hands. The survivor may want to use a relaxation exercise prior to beginning the tactile exploration if he/she is fearful or anxious about the process. Most therapists can design individualized relaxation exercises for their clients. Or you may find various relaxation exercises in books on relaxation and/or stress management.

Exercise #10: "Exploring the body through imagination"

To reduce anxiety about tactile exploration, you may first want to explore your body in your imagination. To complete this exercise, you will want to find a place that is free of distraction and noise. Make sure that you can rest comfortably and relax in the area that you choose.

Position yourself so that you are as comfortable as possible. Close your eyes if you can. If not, allow your eyes to rest in a neutral position. You may find that your eyes will close on their own as you begin the relaxation.

Breathe deeply and as you exhale (breathe out), let go of all the muscles in your head and neck. Allow yourself to breathe normally as you experience the muscles letting go, and becoming warm as the tension moves out of them.

Breathe deeply again. As you exhale, let go of all the muscles in your shoulders, allowing the tension to move off the shoulders and down through the arms and off the fingertips. Breathe normally until you are ready to take another deep breath.

When you are ready, breathe deeply again and as you exhale, let go of all the muscles in your arms, allowing the tension to flow off the arms through the fingertips. Experience the warmth of the muscles as they continue to relax more and more.

Breathe deeply again. Let go of all the stress in the torso, allowing those muscles to relax from the top of your head, down through your neck and shoulders, through your arms, and down through your body. Breathe normally, as you relax and allow your body to be fully supported by the chair in which you are sitting.

Breathe deeply again and allow all of the muscles in your lower body to relax and melt away the tension. Focus now on relaxing all of your body parts. Allow yourself to maintain this relaxation as you use your imagination.

Imagine standing nude in an area that is totally safe and private, where no one can get in and where you are totally secure. Imagine your hands rising to touch your head and hair, smoothing the skin over your face and cupping your jaw. Imagine letting your hands drop to touch your shoulders, then move down to your chest. Imagine your fingers gently stroking your breasts (or pectorals) and nipples. Imagine touching your abdomen then moving your hands down and feeling the texture of your pubic hair and genitalia. Imagine your hands gently probing your genitals, then stroking the skin of your thighs, calves, and feet.

When you have allowed your imagination to work for you, you can take a deep breath and return to your normal state of consciousness. Remember that it is important to maintain your relaxation throughout the imagery, even if that means stopping and starting as many times as you need to. Pace yourself. You have the time.

For many survivors, touching the body is an uncomfortable and shameful process. One way to avoid some of the shameful feelings is to have the survivor first explore his/her body in the shower or bath (if those places are unsafe or generate anxiety, skip this alternative). This way, the survivor can explore during the necessary process of bathing.

Exercise #11: "Tactile exploration"

The next time you're in the bath or shower, try this exercise:

Apply soap to your hands and work up a lather. Then, when you are ready, allow your hands to gently glide over your body, beginning with your neck and shoulders and working your way down to your toes. Move your hands in a circular motion around particularly sensitive areas. There's no need to spend a lot of time in any one area, unless you enjoy it. Allow as much time for this process as you feel comfortable.

As you gain some experience and comfort with this exercise, you can begin to explore areas that have been overly-sensitive or associated with shame or fear. When you can feel relaxed during this process, you can opt to continue with an internal exploration of the vagina and anus. This process must be individualized for each person and it should be approached slowly so that the experience is positive and safe, rather than intrusive and negative.

From this point, you and your partner can opt to explore while bathing or during "dry" private time. Many survivors find that they can relax more easily in a room other than the bedroom, especially if the abuse occurred in a bedroom. Again, it is important that the survivor remain relaxed during the exploration process, and revert back to simpler or safer exercises should he/she begin to experience anxiety, fear or panic. When the survivor has achieved relaxation with tactile exploration, he/she can opt to attempt sexual stimulation. If the survivor has difficulties with sexual arousal, he/she may want to use verbal, auditory, visual, or sensory aids.

Many women become most easily aroused when they read about a safe, sexual interaction. Some survivors may choose the romance novel, and others may opt for a racier version with more explicit sexual details. Men are most frequently aroused by visual stimuli and may choose to look at erotica, either in magazines or on video. Your partner may become aroused by the sound of your voice and may want you to make an audio tape for him/her with selected words, phrases or fantasies that your partner finds stimulating. Finally, many survivors find that arousal is enhanced with the use of sensory aids such as dildoe, vibrators, wool mittens, leather gloves or satin lingerie. During the arousal process, survivors may want to try a combination of aids. Matthew shares his experience as follows:

> *When I began my healing process, I was afraid of really living in my body. You know, I learned to split off from it so well that I didn't know if I could take how it really felt when I connected. I tried some of the exercises, and they were OK. It took a while though! Anyway, the hardest thing for me when I was learning how to, excuse my language jack off, again, was that I didn't like the way my hands felt on my cock. Every time I touched myself, I remembered Neil's hands on my body and I'd instantly lose my erection. I was so afraid and I just didn't want those memories attached to my new sexuality. I read about trying different things, like gloves and stuff. Well, I felt pretty weird about it, but I decided to try it (since I had nothing to lose). I tried wearing leather gloves, but that was even worse, so I tried on a pair of cashmere mittens. You wouldn't believe the effect! My hands, safely entrenched in cashmere felt good on my body and I didn't have any flashbacks or negative feelings. Man, I just got off! Now that I've learned to give myself that pleasure again, I've started getting used to the feeling of my own hands on*

my body and things feel like they're finally getting to be normal.

As has been noted previously, some survivors can manage arousal, but are unable to sustain the arousal or to achieve orgasm. When the survivor is exploring his or her body, the most important concept is that of relaxation. The goal is for the survivor to learn to associate positive feelings with sexuality, rather than just to orgasm. Given that goal, it may benefit the survivor to learn to stay with the process, to experience the sexual stimulation for as long as she or he wishes, rather than for the length of time that it takes to orgasm. Your partner needs to learn to make love to himself or herself rather than simply release her or his body's sexual tension (that can even be accomplished through physical exercise!). If your partner has been able to complete these activities and is still not orgasmic, she or he may want to focus more on the control issues associated with the orgasm.

When your partner is attempting to work toward orgasm, it may be helpful to use soothing phrases and/or sexual aids. If he/she has been able to determine why he/she is afraid to orgasm, he/she can develop a list of soothing phrases to repeat to him/herself during sexual exploration and stimulation. For example, the survivor who fears that she will be too vulnerable during orgasm to fight off a potential perpetrator may wish to calm and relax herself during the sexual stimulation, in addition to choosing a private, safe place in which to masturbate (in a locked room). Phrases such as: "I am an adult and I can take care of my body in this way"; "My body deserves this pleasure"; "I can take care of myself, even when I orgasm"; "The release will be pleasurable and fulfilling"; and "I am the one who chooses to free my body" can help the survivor remain relaxed and drop over the orgasm wall. If your partner is frightened of orgasms alone (because of fear of losing control or having flashbacks), he/she may ask you to be present to help him/her remain relaxed and comfortable.

Exercise #12: "Affirmations and soothing for sexual healing"

Sit in a safe place where you and your partner can talk openly about sex without distractions. Review any sexual activities that you and your partner find difficult. Make a list of phrases that can comfort the survivor when he/she is distressed. Add any phrases or affirmations that may enhance sexual pleasure or intimacy.

Even though the exploration process is designed to be safe, your partner may still experience great discomfort and shame, especially about taking private time to touch and feel his/her own body. Not only may your partner feel guilty for taking private time for something that he/she may consider unimportant (trying to dissociate or deny the body), but he/she may also feel shame and fear about touching his/her body.

Exercise #13: "Places for safe, comfortable sexual exploration"

Sit in a safe place where you and your partner can speak openly about sex without distractions. Make a list of the places where you both feel comfortable using "private time." Where are the places that the survivor feels comfortable and safe, yet you do not feel safe there? Are there places that you can use for personal exploration in which the survivor may not feel comfortable?

Exercise #14: "Solitary masturbation"

When you (either lover or survivor) are ready, let your partner know that you will be taking some private time, and to protect you from any intrusions or distractions. Go to your safe place and initiate relaxation. Some people find music relaxing, while other do not. You may wish to use the relaxation exercise located a few pages back, or another that better suits you. Find a technique that allows you to totally relax your body.

When you are relaxed, allow your hands to lightly touch your sensual areas (those that you find sexually stimulating). Select an area with which you associate the least fear or anxiety. Allow yourself to touch and explore your body for as long as you can feel relaxed. If you are able to remain relaxed long enough to orgasm, good for you! If you are able to stick with it only a few minutes, good for you! Stay with the masturbation only as long as you can remain relaxed and free of fear and anxiety.

Your partner was probably taught during the abuse that he/she was worthless and dirty, and may thus be ashamed of his/her body. He/she may have experienced feelings of guilt, disgust and anger during sexual interaction and may feel unable to divest these emotions from current, safe sexuality. Finally, if your partner has experienced or heard about flashbacks, he/she may fear the onset of flashbacks during the sexual exploration.

It is important to support your partner's attempts at self-exploration; it is also important to face the realities of the process. Sexual exploration of any kind, may indeed, set off flashbacks. Such an experience need not be totally negative or bad. If your partner fears flashbacks and can enlist your support, he/she may be able to engage in the exploration, knowing that you are near should he/she begin to feel out-of-control or unsafe. Should this occur, it is important to keep your partner oriented and safe from harm. Here is an example of such an event:

> *Upon hearing a shriek from the other room, Mike runs to the aid of his wife, Sherri, who has begun a masturbation session minutes before. He enters their bedroom to find her huddled in the corner, hands cradling her head and quivering.*
> *"Sherri, are you OK?"*
> *"Stop it! Stop it! Stop it!"*
> *"Sherri, it's Mike. Sherri, tell me how I can help it stop."*
> *"It hurts. Make it stop. It hurts!"*
> *"Sherri, it's me, Mike. We're here in Tampa in our room in the house we built together. You're safe and I'm here to help you."*
> *"No, get away. Get away. Don't hurt me!"*
> *"Sherri, it's Mike and I would never hurt you. I'm going to sit right over here and talk with you until you can relax and feel safer. Today is the 12th of June and we're in Tampa. You were in here to do an exercise that Dr. de Beixedon gave you to do and you got frightened. I'm here to help you feel*

safer. Can I get something to help you feel more comfortable?"

"I'm afraid he'll hurt me. Make him stop. Get him away from me. He wants to get at me."

"Sherri, it's Mike and I'm the only one in the room with you. I know that he hurt you very badly a long time ago, but he's gone now, and he can't hurt you here. You are thirty-two years old, and you're five foot six and you are no longer a little girl. We can face this together. Remember when we talked about that before we got married?"

"Mike?"

"Yes, Sherri, it's me, Mike. How can I help you feel safe? Would you like to look at me and talk about what happened?"

"Oh, Mike, I'm so afraid. It was happening all over again."

"I bet it felt like it was happening, but you're OK and you're safe. When did the memories come on?"

"I was touching myself, just like the book said, and then I began to feel like someone was watching me, and I started to panic. The more I panicked, the more memories started to flood me."

"Sherri, you're OK now. Touching yourself is OK, and you had the right to be alone and get pleasure. Remember that it's OK to stop when you're anxious, but you're all right now. Do you want to stay here for a while, or what?"

"I don't know. I feel weird."

"Don't push yourself too hard, but if you want to try the exercise again and you'd like my help I'll do whatever I can. Would you feel safer if I sat here and encouraged you?"

Sherri breathes a sigh of relief and giggles, *"I don't think I'm ready for that yet, Mike. Maybe I'll just try some easier exercises for a couple of minutes."*

"Sounds like a great idea. I'll be sitting in the den if you need me. You look a lot more comfortable now. How do you feel?"

"Better. Safer. I'm just going to sit for a while. Can I have my teddy bear?"

"Sure. Call me if you need me."

If your partner has experienced flashbacks (or fears having them), complete the following exercises:

Exercise #15: "Flashback descriptions"

Sit with your partner and review the flashbacks that he/she has already experienced. Encourage the survivor to write about the flashbacks so that the experience is better contained. If the survivor has not yet experienced flashbacks, but fears them, have him/her describe any fears in detail.

Exercise #16: "Managing flashbacks"

Sit with your partner and review the experience that you have had with flashbacks up until this point. Discuss the fears and concerns each of you have about the flashbacks that may occur in the future. Together, develop a set of instructions on how to manage the flashbacks should they occur. Write the instructions down and keep a copies in the areas which will be used for "private time."

Beyond self-exploration and orgasm is a realm in which the survivor may elect to sexually interact with a partner in a sexual alliance. In their book, *Incest and Sexuality*, Maltz and Holman suggest that to ensure that survivors are not abused again and can maintain self-respect and self-esteem within their evolving sexuality, five basic conditions must be met. These conditions are:

C.E.R.T.S. for Positive, Healthy Sexuality

Consent
I can freely and comfortably choose whether or not to engage in sexual activity. I am able to stop the activity at any time during the sexual contact.

Equality
My feeling of personal power is on an equal level with my partner. Neither of us dominates the other.

Respect

I have a positive regard for myself and for my partner. I feel respected by my partner. I feel supportive of my partner and supported by my partner.

Trust

I trust my partner on both a physical and emotional level. We have a mutual acceptance of vulnerability, and an ability to respond to it with sensitivity.

Safety

I feel secure and safe within the sexual setting. I am comfortable with and assertive about where, when, and how the sexual activity takes place. I feel safe from the possibility of unwanted pregnancy and/or sexually transmitted diseases.

You may realize that these conditions are basic requirements for the development of any intimate relationship, but are even more important to the abuse survivor who is developing his/her sexuality. These components are further explored in Chapter 5.

Once these conditions are met, you and your partner may want to try exercises to enhance feelings of trust and safe intimacy. If your partner is just reentering the world of sexual interaction, it may be beneficial for him/her to first learn to interact with you while clothed. One exercise that survivors can do with their partners is the mirroring exercise.

Exercise #17: "Mirroring"

Choose a place that you and your partner can interact without noise or distractions. Sit comfortably, facing one another. In this exercise, you mimic or mirror the behavior of your partner, being careful to stay near him/her without actually touching. For example, if Sherri were to place her hand in the air in front of her face, Mike would raise his hand to the same place, but without touching Sherri's. Be creative with your movement. See how close you can come without violating the personal space of your partner.

The mirroring exercise allows the survivor to feel that his/her actions and space will be respected, while allowing the couple to stay physically close. A modified version of the mirroring exercise is the healthy touch, in which survivors mirror and experience the touch offered by their partners without engaging in overt sexual activity.

Exercise #18: "Healthy touch"

In the healthy touch exercise, you will make physical contact but without intending sexual stimulation. To keep the exercise free of anxiety, review your sexual "zones" with one another, so that these areas can be avoided until future interactions. Find a comfortable place in which to sit, that is free of intrusions and distractions. Sit facing your partner. Whomever chooses to initiate contact, moves a body part and the partner meets it. For example, Mike may offer his hand in midair to Sherri. She would meet his hand, following its motion through the air with her own hand, being careful not to break the bond and steering clear of sexual touch.

Couples may also experience healthy touch through frontal or posterior (back) massage, while clothed or nude.

Exercise #19: "Clothed massage"

Find a flat surface that is cool enough for you and your partner to interact while clothed, without becoming overheated. As massage involves rubbing the body, whomever is going to receive the massage may want to wear light or tightly-fitting clothing. Because this exercise is intended to increase intimacy and relaxation, make sure that the person receiving the massage remains relaxed during the massage—even if it means stopping or starting many times.

The person being massaged lies (face up or face down) on a flat surface. Allow him/her to make this choice, as each individual may respond differently. Beginning at the neck, gently massage the muscles in a circular motion, maintaining contact between your hands and the body at all times. Remember to massage hands and feet, as these body parts are frequently overused and forgotten.

Exercise #20: "Nude massage"

When you and your partner feel prepared, you may choose to do nude massage. The practice is the same as massage while clothed (except for the clothing). Be sure to review with your partner the particularly sensitive areas that he/she may have. Avoid massaging these areas with too much vigor. You may decide to skip these areas or to massage them lightly on your way to another body part. Remember to allow the one being massaged to determine how he/she will lie. Help to maintain optimal relaxation while experimenting with this new form of touch.

When you are able to maintain healthy touch and remain relaxed, you can choose to move on to sexual touch. Again, it is imperative that both of you remain relaxed while engaged in sexual interaction, even if this means stopping one activity and initiating an easier activity. Often couples who are working toward sexual interaction will revert to "imagery" or fantasy exercises when other "tactile" exercises elicit anxiety or fear. An example of an imagery exercise follows.

Exercise #21: "Fantasy creation"

Go to your "safe" place where you are free of distractions and intrusions. Sit together and explore the ideas which each of you find sexually stimulating. Together, develop a sexual fantasy that can promote arousal without fear or anxiety. After the fantasy has been developed, you may wish to write it down. Some people are aroused more easily by reading erotica, while others are aroused by verbally saying it or hearing it.

Exercise #22: "Sharing fantasy"

Once you have completed the exercise above, attempt to use the fantasy, without sexual interaction. Lie together in your safe place, clothed or unclothed, and review your shared fantasy. Allow your bodies to become aroused by the details of the fantasy, but avoid sexual contact.

While some couples may be uncomfortable with the idea, shared masturbation can be a healthy way for a couple to become intimate without the fear often associated with penetration.

Exercise #23: "Shared masturbation"

In shared masturbation, the couple agrees to relax together and possibly develop or use verbal fantasy. Go to your safe place, clothed or partially clothed. Position yourself so that you can see one another—as close together as you are comfortable.

When you are comfortable, allow your hands to glide over areas of your body that you find sexually stimulating and develop the feelings of arousal. It is not necessary for each of you to begin masturbating at the same time; however, it may enhance your interaction as the sexual excitement feeds into the shared fantasy and vice-versa. Masturbate until you have had sufficient enjoyment or until you reach orgasm. Continue relaxing together, touching or remaining separate, depending on what you are comfortable with.

A modified version of shared masturbation is mutual masturbation, in which each member of the couple touches or strokes the other's genitalia for sexual arousal, pleasure or orgasm.

Exercise #24: "Mutual masturbation"

As in shared masturbation, the couple would agree to go to their safe place to relax together, sharing fantasy or perhaps viewing or listening to erotica together. Ask your partner if you can touch him/her, and agree on the area at which each of you will start. When there is agreement, allow your hands to touch or stroke one another.

When you engage in mutual masturbation, it is imperative that you stay connected with one another, frequently asking if your partner would like the touch to stay the same or whether it might be altered for increased pleasure. Each of you can then ask or offer ideas for enhanced pleasure. Continue the activity until sated or until orgasm is achieved. It is unnecessary for each member to orgasm, though mutual orgasm may increase your sense of intimacy and trust.

When you are able to remain relaxed during shared sexual interaction, you may want to attempt different activities or a combination of activities with or without penetration. Continued communication between you and your partner is most important in order that both of you are respected and fulfilled. When your partner decides to attempt penetration with you, communication will need to be in peak form. As penetration is often one of the most common triggers for flashbacks and body memories, you will need to be ready to withdraw should this occur.

The act of intercourse is one of the most difficult to retrain, as it is encompassing and often overwhelming. You may need to put your own needs aside while your partner is learning to enjoy the penetration, and you may have to take care of your own sexual needs separate from the interactions with your partner. You may also witness tears and frustration during the process and will need to continuously check in with your partner to determine whether he/she has reached a stopping point. Again, while exploring together, it is imperative that your partner remain with you and oriented at all times. Most couples benefit from talking before, during, and after they engage in sexual activity because it allows for increased communication, comfort and intimacy.

While some couples attempt to work on sexual healing without the assistance of a counselor, surrogate or therapist, others find it helpful to talk through their issues and obstacles with an objective helper. In addition, some couples find it useful to read about sexual healing exercises, or to view video tapes designed to teach people to become orgasmic. These resources are cited in Chapter 10.

To enhance your sexuality together, it is important that you work together to create a loving and respectful alliance. The following chapter may help you develop the kind of relationship that will allow you to relax and grow, independently and together.

Section II

Developing A Healthy Relationship
With Your Partner

Now you've gotten to know a little bit about your partner as a survivor. You have learned some basics about sexual abuse, and have begun to realize the impacts that the abuse has had on your partner and on you as well. You have probably observed physical, behavioral, emotional and psychological effects in your partner already. You've also started to recognize what your partner did in the past to cope with his/her abuse.

Now it's your turn. The next few chapters will give you an idea of what a healthy relationship is (this may be especially helpful if you grew up in a dysfunctional family), and what you can expect in your current relationship. In order to develop a realistic relationship with your partner, you may have to compromise and accept that the relationship will not be ideal (no real relationship is ever perfect). And, in order to help your partner feel safe enough to trust you and to share his/her life with you, you'll have to learn to be a co-survivor. Taking the steps together can be difficult, but when you get where you're going, it can be wonderful.

Chapter 5
Real vs. Ideal

What is a Healthy Relationship? What are Its Components?

For decades, maybe even centuries, people have been trying to determine what makes for a good relationship. Long ago, in primitive cultures, men hunted, and women gathered and produced children. Many investigators suggest that this division of labor was based in the fact that men were considered expendable, while women were valued for their ability to reproduce, and required protection from the dangers of the wild. Even though women merited asylum, they were not given a choice about sexual orientation, status, position, or partner. Women in these groups were apparently treated as chattel rather than as partners.

As climates became more temperate and large game declined in numbers, agrarian or farming cultures developed. In these societies, power became more balanced as it became apparent that women and men could sow seeds equally well. Women shared in the labor of farming, though they were still at the mercy of the patriarchal society that valued them most as givers of life. As life gained "civilization," partnerships became more common than servility. With the dawn of the industrial age, and the increase in military enlistment, women were able to work at positions previously reserved for men. They gained the vote and became "equal" members of society. Due to the horrible, unregulated conditions of the factories, many women died as a result of accidents and disease. In addition, when wartime ended and soldiers returned home, women were expected to give up their positions and return home to keep house and to bear children. Even during this era, in which women gained power as wage-earners, there was little thought to the components of partnerships, as spouses were frequently away at war.

It took another half-century for women to regain their places in the world of work and to earn comparable wages. It took two more major wars, the massive decline of the extended and nuclear families, and extensive inflation for women to achieve equitable status and the respect of male co-workers and partners. But who's to say, after that intensive struggle that men and women actually seek balance and equality in their intimate relationships? Who's to say that men and women don't still sustain the unbalanced, male-dominated pairings associated with primitive culture? What do men and women want from each other? What kind of relationship facilitates health and growth for each member of the couple and how can lovers and survivors get there together?

Components of A Healthy Relationship

In her best-selling book, *Struggle for Intimacy*, Janet Woititz posits that a healthy relationship promotes the existence of an environment where "I can be me. You can be you. We can be us. I can grow. You can grow. We can grow together."[10] The premise has appeal: each party can be independent, and still develop unity. Each partner has equal status and similar goals.

Other investigators have also suggested that relationships which are based on independence and similarity have the potential for durability and longevity while relationships developed in complimentary tend to be passionate and short-lived. In other words, if the partners are mirror images of one another (e.g. hot/cold, conservative/liberal), the attraction may be intense.

Neither can really know what the other is feeling, but is drawn to that individual who complements him/her so well. So often the media offers us examples of the country boy turned metropolitan with the help of his urban and jet-set partner. Unfortunately, while the complementary makes for passion and excitement, it generally does not provide enough of the components for long-lasting intimacy and romance. What are the components of those independent, yet fruitful, pairings which allow growth, development, health and happiness?

For intimacy and enduring bonds to develop in a relationship, there are a number of conditions and qualities that must be developed, nourished, and maintained. The most significant include, but are not limited to: individuality, acceptance, communication, honesty, respect, trust, vulnerability, mutual sexual interaction, empathy, consideration, compassion, understanding, and congruence.

Individuality

Individuality refers to the process by which a person develops a sense of self and maintains him/herself as a separate but interactive individual. More simply, individuality allows the person to be independent but connected. For most, the process of developing a sense of self takes a lifetime. After adolescence, we have all developed our identities to some degree. When we enter intimate relationships, we often begin to forget who we are in response to our partner's needs and desires and to the synergism which occurs within the partnership. In order to maintain our personalities and meet our own needs, it is important that we develop and maintain both personal and relational boundaries.

In Chapter 2, Gail recounted how her personal boundaries had been consistently crossed by her sexually abusive father. After a time, she became hypovigilant and lost her sense of boundaries with other people. She was constantly bumped, elbowed, and jostled around, because she no longer recognized her right to have personal space around her. In a relationship, Gail would likely deny her right to privacy and personal boundaries and would potentially be re-victimized by intrusive partners who did not bring with them an inherent sense of respect for others. To avoid feelings that are often associated with abuse and violation, each partner needs to gain a sense for how much space, privacy, and separateness he/she needs for himself/herself. It is the responsibility of each partner to maintain those boundaries so that his/her needs are met, but if they agree, partners may assist one another with boundary management.

Personal boundaries allow the individual to relate to his/her partner in a healthier, independent fashion. If each partner can maintain a separate but interactive self, and the couple can agree to some relational boundaries, the partners can avoid co-dependency, enmeshment, and role confusion. It is the responsibility of the couple to decide how they will interact with one another, whom they will include in their relationship, and the degree to which they will relate to others.

Co-dependency refers to the process by which an individual believes that his/her sense of worth depends on the happiness or success of his/her partner. Betty, a survivor who married a car salesman (also a survivor), recalls her struggles with co-dependency:

> *When I was growing up our house was always dirty because my mother was never home. I decided that when I married Jacob, I would stay*

at home and keep a lovely house and raise healthy, happy children. Well, after six years of marriage, we found out that we couldn't have children, as my uterus had been so badly damaged during those years of abuse. We were devastated, but I decided to become the best help-mate a man could want. I cooked and cleaned and kept up with the car sales stats every month, but it never really seemed to be good enough. Jacob would come home unhappy, and it no longer mattered what I'd done that day or felt good about. I tried to help him feel better every way I knew, but if nothing worked, I would become distressed and angry at myself. I was responsible for one thing: keeping my husband happy, and I couldn't even do that right.

In her marriage, Betty thought little of her own needs, most likely because her abuser taught her that her needs were unimportant, and that her only function was to meet the needs and desires of the perpetrator. Without intervention, Betty might have maintained her co-dependency and relinquished all sense of self to her husband.

Another dynamic that may develop in a relationship in which the partners fail to maintain personal and relational boundaries is enmeshment. Very often, in families in which abuse occurs, members are thoroughly entrenched in one another's private lives. When a survivor from one of these incestuous families enters a relationship, his/her lack of experience with boundary management may lead to enmeshment in the partner's personal life.

For example, Cary, who was molested by his resident aunt for a number of years, married Lila, and found himself becoming more and more involved in her personal life the longer they were together. At first, he was interested in her routine at work, asking her daily about the things she did, the people with whom she spoke, the places she had driven. Then, Cary became more intrusive into her personal style, asking her about what she would eat, wear, and use. Finally, when Cary began to come to her work to speak with her colleagues in order to "get closer to her," Lila became enraged and asked Cary to seek counseling.

In Cary's case, he learned this enmeshed style of relating from his family of origin. For many other survivors, enmeshment may evolve due to the need for closeness and acceptance without regard for the personal boundaries set by others.

Role confusion may also result from the failure to maintain personal or relational boundaries. One couple relates their story:

> *Dan: After I lost my job, I got pretty depressed and didn't really do much. I spent a lot of time hanging around the house and I lost a sense of who I was. I didn't have many boundaries, because I felt like I was a failure and that I didn't deserve any.*

> *Bea: I think that even before Dan lost his job, I had grown frustrated with him and with our life together, but I just didn't do anything about how I felt. I figured we'd work it out somehow.*

> *Dan: I think that I had some idea that Bea felt that way, because when I finally felt up to doing things, I began to do stuff for her. Like, first it was doing yard work and stuff to keep me busy, and then it was other chores so that the house would be clean when she got home from work, then it would be little personal things for her.*

> *Bea: I was pulling the weight for us financially, and I was exhausted. When Dan started to get off his butt, I was pretty thankful. I figured that at least he was doing something other than watching football. When he started doing more for me, who was I to say, "no."*

> *Dan: After a while, I didn't do anything for myself anymore, and I spent all of my time involved with the house and her. I didn't have any friends, hobbies or a job. I started to lose all sense of me in the relationship.*

Bea: It never occurred to me that Dan was unhappy about his role in the relationship. I mean it never even occurred to me that he'd lost it. I was just enjoying being treated well. Who needs a husband anyway?

Dan: I really woke up one day when one of our neighbors saw me trimming Bea's hair in the backyard. He came right over and asked me if I'd like to be his wife too. All of the sudden I realized I had no idea who I'd become.

Sometimes role confusion can exist for both partners, especially if both have a difficult time maintaining relational boundaries.

Acceptance

In addition to the development and maintenance of healthy personal and relational boundaries, acceptance, of both oneself and one's partner, is a prerequisite for any intimate relationship. Acceptance of self includes the recognition of one's strengths and deficits, of one's values, beliefs and opinions, and of one's feelings and thoughts. It refers to the acceptance of responsibility for the feelings one has, the actions one takes and the consequences one must manage. It means that when all things are considered, the individual can accept who she/he is and what she/he does.

As much as acceptance of self refers to taking responsibility for who one is and what one does, acceptance of another refers to not taking responsibility for the other person's feelings, thoughts and actions. Accepting your partner's quirks, habits, and style doesn't mean that you agree with what she/he does or says, it means that you accept their right to be separate and equal. Joy shares insight that was a long time in coming:

Ron and I used to go out to parties and have a really nice time, UNTIL Ron would start cutting up. He would make these remarks and jokes that I found so embarrassing. I used to think I was going to die of shame and I would do everything I could think of to get him to stop, or to go home with me. And he used to just laugh it up even more then. I used to think, "Oh, well, another friend lost,

*another home we can't return to." As I got a little
older (and had a little more therapy!), I started to
recognize that Ron was his own person, and that
I was not responsible for his behavior. He was.
And if he wasn't ashamed of what he did, and he
didn't have any adverse consequences to deal with
(that affected me), then what he did was his
business, and I had to accept him as is or get out.*

Sometimes, survivors find that acceptance of their partners
is one of the hardest tasks, because it requires that survivors
agree to stop trying to control their partners. It means that
sometimes, the survivor may feel helpless in the face of his/her
partner's behavior, as the survivor recognizes that she/he cannot
change or control the partner's actions, thoughts or feelings. If
the survivor can manage his/her own feelings, and agree to accept
those feelings that arise (whatever they might be), then the
survivor can learn to accept the partner.

Honesty
Sometimes, acceptance hinges on the honesty of both
partners. In order to be honest with someone else, it is
imperative that the individual be honest with him/herself. It is
so easy to lie to ourselves and to "snow white" the truth, so
that we don't have to face the hard stuff. It is so much easier to
accept, if we only need to accept the positive. It is often much
more difficult to recognize and own up to the negative realities
that may be part of our current and past lives. Some individuals
(survivors often fall into this group) find it easier to accept the
negatives and balk against accepting the positive aspects of their
lives or pleasant qualities that they possess.

They are brutally honest, but fail to see the beauty on the
other face of the coin. These individuals are often trained by
their families and partners to believe that they are worth very
little, and that they are incapable of succeeding. As a result,
these individuals accept negative qualities and characteristics
as "normal," while they have difficulty believing or accepting
their positive features (as they have little experience or training
with these ideas or concepts). In this case, the individual must
become much more comprehensively honest with him/herself
before she/he can be truly honest in the partnership.

When both parties are able to be honest with themselves, they can learn to be honest with each other. Relationships are generally simplified by honesty, as no webs are woven to cover up deceptions. Honesty within the relationship allows each partner to feel respected by the other, even when the truth may be difficult to swallow. Honesty may not be the easiest route to take in the relationship but it is the path which generally promotes growth, health and happiness.

Respect

As a person begins to achieve an honest perspective of himself or herself and others, he or she can develop respect for self and others. An individual who develops respect for oneself learns that positive qualities and actions increase a sense of self-esteem. This esteem inhibits an individual from putting oneself at risk, and is a reminder that he or she is worth protecting.

As stated previously, respect for another's opinions, thoughts, or feelings does not require one to agree to those, or to accept them as one's own, it simply means that one can agree to allow another individual to be separate and equal. When the choices or opinions of another concur with one's own thoughts and values, respect may incorporate feelings of admiration and esteem for the other.

Consideration

When an individual respects his or her partner, he or she is considerate of the partner's beliefs, interests, values, needs, desires, and goals (to name a few things); and tries to avoid putting the partner down, making fun of him or her, or minimizing his or her importance.

Consideration refers to the honest attention paid to oneself and to others. This careful thought of one's own position and the position held by others must be honest, while at the same time, should not be intentionally harmful or hurtful.

Communication

One way that couples can learn to be considerate of one another's needs, desires, thoughts and feelings is through open, honest, assertive communication. Clear communication permits each party to maintain his/her own opinions and thoughts and to share them with another who agrees to respect them.

Additionally, communication between the partners can promote understanding (both within each individual and between the partners).

Communication can be passive, assertive or aggressive. Passive communication refers to the process in which the needs and desires of one party are sacrificed for the needs and desires of the other. For instance, when John asks Delia which movie she would like to see, Delia responds passively, "Oh, I'll see whatever you're interested in, John."

Aggressive communication occurs when the needs of one person are disregarded for the needs or desires of another. In this case, John might tell Delia which movie they will see, despite her requests that they see a different type of film. With an aggressive style, John is not sensitive to Delia's issues or interests; instead, he is absorbed in his own thoughts and feelings. In both passive and aggressive styles of communication, someone generally gets hurt, whether intentionally or unintentionally.

Sometimes, when the individual responds passively, he or she has a hidden wish that goes unexpressed. When that need or desire is not fulfilled, the individual may become resentful of his or her partner and may act out that resentment in subtle ways. An example of passive-aggressive communication follows:

> *Delia has been home all day with the kids and is hoping that John will come home and take her out to dinner. John returns home and asks Delia if she has any special plans for the evening. She tells him that she does not and he suggests that they stay home to eat and watch a video. Delia, looking forward to leaving the house for once (but never having told John of her wishes), burns the dinner, and "forgets" to pick up the video, disrupting John's plans for a quiet evening at home (and probably providing all of the components for an argument later, in which she can vent her anger at John for being insensitive to her needs as a wife and woman).*

Assertive communication allows each party to express his or her opinions, thoughts and feelings, and have them respected by the other. No one's needs are intentionally disregarded or minimized. When John and Delia communicate assertively, each is able to express his or her interests without fear of harassment or insult. The ensuing decision is a combination or compromise of the wishes of each partner. In assertive communication, there are no sensory mismatches. For more information regarding sensory mismatching in non-assertive communication, see the Informational Highlight below.

Informational Highlight
Sensory mismatching

Whenever Delia makes a verbal statement, it is accompanied by appropriate visual cues. When she is angry at John for being insensitive, she may frown, clench her jaw, and furrow her eyebrows. When John is glad to see Delia at the end of his day, he smiles and opens his arms to her.

Sensory mismatches occur when one form of communication is accompanied by an inappropriate, unexpected or mismatched form of communication. When Delia says, "Oh, sure... it's fine if we stay home," she she may be thinking, "No, I want to get out of this house!" She may avert her eyes, frown, and put an edge to the tone of her voice. She may even assume a more aggressive posture, such as straightening her back, holding her head stiffly, and placing her hands on her hips.

Research suggests that most impressions are formed from visual rather than verbal information. If Delia acts with hostility, while she is making a verbally passive response, John may catch on to her frustration. If John is scowling when he opens his arms to Delia as he enters the house, she is certain to experience some confusion.

If she is like many partners, especially those that are survivors, she may think, "What did I do wrong, now?" rather than, "I wonder what his problem is?" To keep the relationship healthy and happy, communication must be consistent, honest, and assertive.

Trust

When the relationship promotes individuality, acceptance, honesty, respect, consideration and assertive communication, it will also likely enhance trust between the partners. As with acceptance and respect, the individual must first learn to trust him/herself before real trust can be invested in a partner. In order to trust oneself, one must know one's boundaries and be able to predict one's behavior.

Trust develops from understanding and accepting one's values, beliefs, feelings, and position in the world. Self-esteem can cultivate trust in one's self. When an individual feels that she or he can trust her/himself, she or he can feel free to interact with a partner without fearing the loss of identity. The trust that is developed between two people can allow them to become vulnerable with one another, to reveal their true selves and to be affected by one another.

Since trust has the potential to vastly impact partners, it must be earned. So often, adults who have grown up with unpredictable, alcoholic or abusive parents perceive trust in an all-or-nothing vein: either they are unable to trust at all in a relationship, or they invest all of their trust with those who have not yet earned it. Children who grow up in abusive or negligent homes are not provided with role models who can teach them about trust, so when they enter relationships as adults, they have little understanding of what trust involves. They will approach the quandary optimistically ("Everyone is trustworthy, until proven not." These folks get hurt often) or pessimistically ("No one is trustworthy." These people are lonely and isolated because they fear connection with others so much that they fail to interact at all).

Upon entering a relationship, survivors are apt to go to those extremes. Some survivors test their partners again and again, but partners are never able to truly pass the tests. This testing may frustrate and enrage you. Sometimes, awareness of your partner's desire to learn to trust can assuage these angry and difficult feelings. After all, your partner wouldn't be "testing" if she or he were not working on "trusting!" Sexual abuse forces the survivor to believe that those who come close will hurt, so even if the partner passes the test, the survivor may conclude that she or he has not yet developed a challenging or accurate enough test!

For other survivors, the need to attain intimacy and affection is so great that they will take whatever they can get. They may not bother to test a partner's trust-worthiness prior to making an emotional commitment. Unfortunately, this leaves the survivor vulnerable to abuse and exploitation by others.

It is important that potential partners develop trust in one another over a period of time. Lovers and survivors must learn to open small windows to their spirits and to share those tiny parts of themselves freely, leaving themselves open to the impacts of one another. If potential partners take advantage of that vulnerability or cause harm, then retreat and reconsideration may be imperative. In the event that the potential partner treats those opportunities to really see the individual with respect and compassion, the individual learns that sharing can be positive and can invest even further.

Vulnerability

Physical and emotional vulnerability are some of the hardest components of intimacy to achieve in a relationship. It requires trust, strength, and risk from both partners and demands that control be shared rather than placed within one individual or the other. It means agreeing to be open to the impact that another person may have on one's life and being. In the last chapter, Alice related how she was unable to really be vulnerable with her partner. Because of Alice's fear that if she relinquished control she would be abused or destroyed, she was unable to achieve orgasm with her partner. Increased vulnerability, although it felt dangerous to Alice, may have allowed her to interact with her partner more fully and would have allowed Alice a greater degree of input and experience from her partner and from herself.

Mutual Sexual Interaction

As was the case with Alice, vulnerability is often most limited in sexual interaction. Yet, mutual sexual interaction can provide some of the best nourishment, play, and replenishment that a committed relationship can offer. What needs to happen for sexual interaction and vulnerability to coincide and potentiate one another?

In Chapter 4, it was suggested that five basic conditions need to exist between two individuals for a healthy sexual relationship to develop. These include consent, equality, respect, trust and safety—all of which are required for the creation of intimacy between partners. For the promotion of healthy sexuality, partners must be compatible on a number of different levels.

Sexual orientations must be compatible, although they may not be the same. For instance, many bisexual women become involved with lesbian women and with heterosexual men. (They rarely date only other bisexual women.) Similarly, bisexual men may have both heterosexual and homosexual partners.

Secondly, both partners must be aware of the level of sexual emergence of their partner and this must be in accordance with the desires of each person. Some individuals may want to be sexually involved with others who have more sexual experience. Other couples want to have comparable levels of experience.

In a related arena, the sexual interests of the couple must be equitable. This means that the types of sexual interactions, degree of involvement, and use of sexual enhancement aids must be agreed upon prior to the sexual interaction. For most couples, sexual exploration and creativity synergize with the intimacy already present in the relationship—and it certainly adds to the fun and passion. For a sexual abuse survivor and his/her partner sexual "surprises" may result in more negative rather than positive feelings and experiences.

Finally, partners must agree on rules and boundaries of their sexual relationship for sexual activity to be healthy and nourishing. The following vignette highlights some of these concerns:

> We started dating a little over two years ago, and we've really been through a lot together. It took us a while to really get in sync with one another, learning about each other's habits, likes, dislikes. We learned this stuff through trial and error, and for the most part that was OK. One thing that was a little tough for us was agreeing on who could be in the relationship. Now, I love women, don't get me wrong, and I love fantasy, but one afternoon when we're laying in bed, Kathy starts talking about how gorgeous her girlfriend is and how she'd like to get it on with her. Well, I got pretty hot thinking about the two of them going at each other, but then, a couple days later, Kathy

brings it up again, and says she's going to invite Carla over. All of the sudden, I started to panic. I went limp and felt nauseous, and I thought I was going to lose it. I got mad, which was the wrong thing to do, but I couldn't keep myself in control. After I thought about it for a while, I apologized, and went back to explain to Kathy about my babysitter. I told her that Christine had always made me feel that I had to satisfy her every wish, with whomever she desired. I remembered, then, about the others I had been with, and the shame that I felt. The thought of being in bed with Kathy and having to please someone else as well, felt just like that sick, obligated sex that I endured for so long as a kid. It took Kathy and me a while, but we've gotten past that day, and we've generated a lot of sexual creativity that's OK for both of us.

Because adults often forget how to play, or "grow out of" play, life can become pretty grim for those over age ten. In order to keep relationships alive, there must be opportunity for play. Sexual interaction is one of the "accepted" arenas for play between adults. This being the case, it is important that couples invest energy in developing trust with one another, so that they can be vulnerable and share with one another freely. As the couple learns to trust and share more openly, the avenues for creative sexual play increase exponentially and the fear, shame and embarrassment which may have previously existed for sexual fantasy and interaction can be released.

In addition to the components already noted, healthy relationships require the presence of empathy and compassion, two skills which can be honed as one learns to accept and understand oneself and one's partner.

Empathy

Empathy must exist for oneself as well as for one's partner. Empathy for self may involve looking at a part of oneself and allowing emotions to surface and be accepted. For example, many clinicians believe that it is important for the survivor to get in touch with the abused child that she or he has hidden inside.

Learning to listen to that distressed inner child may allow the survivor to feel sadness and to nurture that part of him/herself in a way that no one else can.

Learning to empathize with another individual involves taking his/her perspective for the purpose of experiencing and being sensitive to the emotions associated with that perspective. For example, one of the women who is most dear to me is African-American, and as much as I want to understand what is like to walk around in her skin, I cannot. When I want to empathize with her during her trials and tribulations, I search for that part of me which has been oppressed by others, the part which has been unacceptable to others, that part which has met with resistance and fear, that part which has made me different. And when I reach up and take hold of that part, I can experience emotions which may resemble her own, and I can empathize with her, even if I'll never know what it's really like. In a similar way, there are many counselors who work with abuse survivors, who were lucky enough to have avoided abuse themselves. And while they may not have shared the abuse experience, they can identify with the pain experienced by their clients and patients, and provide empathy for the horror that the survivor has endured. The empathy, the feeling that someone else is willing to "try out" one's experience, and to remain, though his/her instinct may be to run and hide, can be incredibly therapeutic. I recall one of the simplest and most intensely rewarding sentences that I ever heard:

> *A survivor and I had been working together for some months and I was trying everything I could think of so that she could feel safe enough to talk about her abuse with me. One day, things must have seemed more secure and nurturing to her and she told me one of the most gruesome tales I had ever heard. As she finished, she looked up, somehow amazed, and said, "You're still here!"*

When shame and emotional pain are overwhelming, the idea that someone is willing to walk around in your shoes for even a moment, in order to get closer to you and to help ease your pain, is often more rewarding than the most expensive material gift.

Compassion

Compassion, much like empathy, allows the individual to become more nurturing to self and others. Compassion refers to the experience of emotions which power acts of assistance, concern, and love. Self-compassion involves the forgiveness of one's ill-fated experiences, decisions and choices. Self-compassion is exemplified by the survivor who learns to nurture that devastated, abused inner child and to say, "I'm sorry this happened to you. It wasn't your fault." Self-compassion allows the individual to release guilt and the sense of self-blame that often accompanies child sexual abuse.

Acts of compassion for self allow the survivor to treat himself or herself as valuable and worthwhile, to accept himself or herself for who she or he is and has been. When an individual is able to be compassionate toward oneself, he or she can extend compassion to others. Compassion for another requires an individual to offer mercy or clemency, if not love and acceptance to the one who is suffering. It refers to the act of offering one's unconditional acceptance of another human being, because she or he is human and desires to connect. In the partnership, compassion is a particularly important element in the regeneration of the relationship following personal traumas and relational conflicts.

Congruence

When a relationship has all of these qualities and attributes, it has a greater chance of enduring bad times and good. And, given some congruence, or mutual interests, desires, values and beliefs, this kind of relationship can promote health and happiness over the ages, and adapt to the transitions and counter transitions that both partners experience.

Why is it that frequently, relationships between lovers and survivors are not experienced by either party as healthy, happy, stable, or nurturing? What is it about this particular intimate combination that makes these relationships more difficult than others? What do partners and survivors have to say about one another in terms of their capacity to relate to one another? What kinds of questions are raised about lovers and survivors interrelating with one another? Some of these questions and issues are addressed in the next two chapters.

Exercise #25: "Components of my relationship"

Find a quiet place in which you are safe to think about your relationship. Begin to explore these questions:

> Which of the relationship components explored throughout this chapter are already present in your relationship?
>
> Which are missing?
>
> Have any of them been particularly difficult for you to achieve?

Chapter 6
Modifying Your Love Relationship
For Health and Healing

How are Love Relationships Uniquely Impacted by Sexual Abuse Survival?

Lovers and survivors come together...somehow. And, when they do, for whatever purpose, they face the music of creating a relationship in the throes of passion and despair. Lovers and survivors come together to experience something special, as most couples do, but they generally come to the relationship without the resources which they will need to grow and develop as a unit. It is not that they are unequipped, or that either partner is disabled, it is instead that they are not prepared *individually* to cope with that which arises *relationally*.

The dynamics and issues of the couple in which one or both of them is a survivor are markedly different than the pairing of non-survivors. Thus far, this book has informed you about sexual abuse and its impacts on physical, emotional, psychological and sexual functioning. And, you are now acquainted with the components required for a healthy relationship based on intimacy and honesty. You may be wondering, "What does this mean for me?" or "How can this book help me?"

What follows are some issues and ideas which may help you to better understand your partner and how she or he interacts with you. You may want to assess the current or potential functioning of your relationship as you read through these sections. To make the task simpler, the prerequisites set forth in the previous chapter are addressed in order.

Each of these areas is affected by your partner's survival from sexual abuse. You may find it difficult to recognize that all levels of the relationship will be impacted by your partner's past history of sexual abuse. However, there is hope. Learning how to love a survivor may take some effort but the results of both of your labors can generate deep and enduring intimacy. Read on to explore the effects which sexual abuse may have on the relationship that you have developed with your partner. It may help to make notes on the concepts you can see at work in your own relationship.

"Who Am I?"

In the last chapter, I suggested that in order to develop intimacy in your relationship, it is important for each partner to be himself or herself and to be accepted on that basis. The problem with this idea when it is applied to survivors is that, frequently, survivors feel as if they do not really know who they are—especially if they have sought counseling many years after the abuse has occurred. In these cases, survivors may believe that they have been living a lie, playing out the abuse every day in some way.

Most survivors radically changed their lives and personalities to manage the abuse they endured. The abuser most likely taught the survivor that she or he did not matter, and that the purpose of the survivor's life was to please and serve the perpetrator. As a result of this mental training, the survivor loses sight of her or his original personality, and begins to develop a character consistent with that which the perpetrator requires. As the perpetrator manipulates the survivor into silence, the survivor loses the opportunity to engage with others and to maintain the last shred of the original self.

Survivors learn how to hide—to physically and psychologically escape or avoid the abuse, and to deny the reality of the abuse after its cessation. Because the survivor spends his/her life hiding, he or she knows little of healthy interaction, and is unable to recognize his/her potential. The survivor rarely takes the chance to find out who he or she is. Unfortunately, if the survivor does not explore and develop a healthy sense of self, he or she is left with the psychic remnants left by the perpetrator.

Most likely the survivor will not like who he or she has become as a result of the sexual abuse, and may want to steer clear of relationships in which he or she is free to be himself or herself. Growth within or with another person may seem impossible to the survivor.

The survivor may continue to hide and to isolate. He or she may choose to avoid intimate relationships completely, or may enter relationships which resemble that with the abuser. If the survivor is able to enter a healthy relationship, he or she may begin to recognize old behaviors and feelings, and he or she may do whatever is necessary to terminate, modify, or aggravate the relationship in order to manage the affective chaos fomented by the interpersonal interaction. Lottie's story is good example:

In my heart, there was so much rage, so much disgust for what they had done to me. I used to tell myself that I was going to be different, I was going to be the real me, not what anyone else ordered me to be. And when I met Trevor, I thought I was going to get my chance to be myself, to be loved and accepted for who I was. The closer we got, the stranger I started acting. After a while, I was this hellcat slut, debasing myself left and right, submitting to his every whim, without regard for any of my own wishes or desires. Somehow, I forgot to be me, I kind of forgot that there was a "me" at all. I wanted to die. I just didn't know how to stop being this other person. I wasn't split or anything... (I definitely didn't pull a Sybil, but I felt out of control anyway). It helped when my therapist reminded me that the abuse had started during the early development of my personality. The character I knew as me was this abused child who submitted to every demand to stay alive. Now that I'm safe, I have to figure out who I want to be, and then I have to learn to be that way.

Lottie emphasizes how awful it felt to submit and to debase herself, but she also noted how difficult it was to be any other way. When a survivor has little idea of who she or he is, old behavior learned during the abuse will resurface again and again until it is replaced with new behavior. In order for that transition to occur, the survivor must want to change the behavior, and the old behavior must no longer be reinforced. For example, if Lottie acts submissively and her partner takes advantage of her (repeating the cycle of old abuse), she will continue to submit. If she chooses to learn a new style of responding, and her partner is willing to assist her, the pattern can be changed. This time, when Lottie responds submissively, her partner can choose to ignore the submission and ask that Lottie assert her own needs, providing her with an opportunity to rewrite the old (abusive) script.

In addition to rewriting life scripts, the survivor needs to explore his/her beliefs, values, morals and desires. Those which are healthy and positive are maintained, and those that are not helpful, are excised and replaced. Exploration and growth requires tremendous energy on the part of the survivor and patience and creativity on the part of the partner. Both must agree to the exploration and transformation for the process to be supportive and for the results to be enduring. As the survivor formulates his/her new identity, acceptance of his/her qualities and characteristics can increase. Acceptance of one's partner is an outgrowth of acceptance of the self.

Exercise #26: "Self-portrait"

Take ten minutes and write down a profile of yourself. If you are uncomfortable with writing, try drawing a self-portrait. Remember, this is not going to be graded so go ahead and have fun while you learn about how you see yourself.

"Where do I end and where do you begin?"

Emotional depth and longevity in a relationship require that each partner is his or her own person. For two people to develop intimacy in their relationship, two personalities and selves must exist. Individuality requires that each party agree to be separate from the other, and to respect personal boundaries. Yet, as you may remember from Gail's story, survivors often loose their sense of personal boundaries, and may wander through their relationships wondering, "Where do I stop? Where does my partner begin?"

Fossum & Mason shed some light on the concept of boundaries with their analogy of the "zipper to the self." Children who are raised in families which respect privacy and personal space learn to control their own boundaries. If a child recognizes that his/her body and inner workings belong only to him/her, he/she may imagine that a zipper located outside his/her body has a tag on the inside (to provide maximal control over the child's input and output). These children learn that unless they invite others into their private spaces by "pulling their zippers down," others do not have the right to invade them. These children recognize their rights to protect their bodies and to maintain their privacy. Some researchers describe these children as having internal loci of control. These children have the sense that they can have an impact in their own lives and control what happens to them.

Other children are taught by their families and their abusers that they do not have the right to personal space or privacy. These children are described as having their zipper tags on the outside, so that others can invade the bodies and personal lives of the children whenever they wish. These children quickly learn that they do not have rights to their own boundaries, and they begin to perceive themselves as objects. Their boundaries are generally not respected and maintained, and after some time, these children fail to expect any privacy or respect. They stop making efforts to maintain their personal boundaries, and may not regain this skill unless interventions are made in their behalf (i.e. until they are taught to control their own zippers). These children maintain external loci of control. They believe that their lives and actions are impacted or controlled by others rather than themselves.

It is fairly obvious that survivors of sexual abuse have often been trained to believe that their zipper tags exist outside of themselves, leaving them vulnerable to the aggression and sadism of others. When survivors interact with others, they may find themselves bombarded with stimuli that they feel they have little control over. They may be uncertain how to engage with others in non-abusive situations, and may feel intimidated by others who try to get close to them. Often survivors whose boundaries are weak or non-existent enter familiar, abusive relationships because they understand how to respond to these kinds of partners.

When survivors enter healthy relationships, it is likely that they will feel unsure about themselves, and may attempt to merge with their partners. If survivors do not sense their own boundaries, they may use their partners' boundaries to calm or soothe themselves. If the partner has been raised in a highly enmeshed family, this merging may feel familiar and the partner may concede to it. If the partner has developed healthy personal boundaries, the merging may be experienced as overwhelming, smothering, and even frightening.

For the relationship to flourish, both the survivor and the partner need to develop and maintain good personal boundaries. Again, this means that each person exists as a separate entity with the right to decide who she/he is, how she/he behaves, how much personal space and privacy she/he requires, who her/his partners are, and what roles she/he takes within and outside the relationship. Gail, for example, would have to decide to really be in her body, and to demand that others provide her with sufficient space to exist and move. Gail's boundaries could be improved if she were to become more sensitive to her own body, experiencing its shape and movement. Gail might improve her sense of personal and relational boundaries by surveying and observing others and their maintenance of personal space. As Gail learns to own her body more, she can learn assertiveness skills to maintain her boundaries more effectively. Once Gail becomes more comfortable asserting her rights to privacy and individuality, she can relax and experiment with the structure and strength of her boundaries, and allow them to be more flexible and adaptive within her intimate relationships. Her internal locus of control can allow her to adapt and flexibly react to her external surroundings.

Exercise #27: "Boundaries"

Review the boundaries that you maintain for yourself. How are they like or unlike your partner's personal boundaries? How do you promote or negate relational boundaries?

"How could you love *me*?"

As the survivor grows up in an abusive home, he/she learns denial, deception and self-disdain rather than honesty. Early on, the survivor is taught that the abuse is a secret, and that to tell would be life-threatening. And, if the perpetrator didn't threaten the survivor with his/her own life, you can bet that the abuser threatened to hurt the child's siblings, parents, or pets. Sometimes, the perpetrator doesn't even need to use blatant threat, but may more subtly intimidate the survivor. The abuser may make the survivor believe that others will abandon or reject the survivor if they find out about the abuse. Even the size discrepancy between perpetrator and child victim may threaten the child or adolescent. In many ways, the perpetrator intimidates the survivor into believing that deception and silence are the only options.

As Shakespeare so aptly put it, "Oh, what a tangled web we weave when first we practice to deceive." The lies and deceptions become more and more intricate as the survivor tries to hide the abuse for his/her own survival, as does the abuser for his/her own security. But the lies increase in number and size as everyone tries to hide from the reality of the abuse. In the end, the survivor must either face the abusive reality or turn to more primitive coping strategies, such as denial and dissociation, in order to continue lying. For some survivors, deception is more acceptable than the recognition of abuse.

In addition to the web of lies so pervasive in the abusive family, there is likely to be rampant self-disdain among family members. While some perpetrators think nothing of their abusive behavior, others drown in guilt, shame and self-hatred. While some parents believe that their children deserve the abuse, others own the responsibility and shame for not protecting their children. While some siblings feel lucky to have survived unscathed, others wonder, "Why not me, too?" All of these members of the family experience a range of self-esteem and self-love. On the other hand, the survivor never escapes the shame, guilt and self-hatred generated by the abuse.

In most circumstances of abuse, the perpetrator leads the survivor to believe that he/she is bad, unworthy of better treatment, shameful, in need of punishment, or simply a sexual object without boundaries or desires of his/her own. In other, less common, situations, the perpetrator trains the survivor to believe that the abuse is an expression of love, caring, nurturing and concern. In this situation, the survivor may be left with feelings of helplessness, confusion, and blind loyalty, as was Emily in Chapter 2. In that case, as well as many others, the survivor is more likely to assume responsibility for the abuse, and may not be able to recognize the perpetrator's abuse of power.

In this situation, the survivor blames him- or herself and develops self-disdain and self-hatred in response to over-whelming shame. Even when the survivor gains emotional health over time, these old self-images and feelings may be reflected in an inability to recognize accomplishments and positive qualities, and through a penchant for self-criticism.

For the survivor, honesty rarely liberates or soothes. Instead, honesty is brutal and judgmental, and rarely leaves the survivor with positive feelings for him- or herself. And when survivors attempt to be honest with others, they often find that it is uncomfortable and unfamiliar (because they have so little experience with honesty).

As honesty is a prerequisite for the growth of intimacy in a relationship, survivors may dodge intimate relationships in which they might actually have to face the truth. As the survivor becomes more able to recognize the reality of his/her past, he/she may become more comfortable sharing true feelings, thoughts, and memories with a partner. The development of the "true self" may take time, and the partner may need to assist the survivor in his/her efforts to maintain a stable, realistic self-perception which promotes self-esteem, competence and confidence.

Exercise #28: "Sharing secrets, making disclosures"

If you and your partner feel ready to experiment and communicate, try the following exercise:

Each partner takes five minutes to make a short list of personal "realities." Then, take turns sharing these personal events with one another. Try disclosing less significant or intense realities first, then try more challenging disclosures of honesty.

"What do I deserve?"

Those individuals who have been sexually abused as children and adolescents were treated as faceless objects by their perpetrators. Their privacy and their bodies were invaded shamelessly by men and women who sought to satisfy their own primitive needs and desires. These abusers did not respect the children that they used, but instead focused on each child's ability to serve, and to provide pleasure to the abuser. This lack of respect for the child's personal boundaries, desires, and rights impacts the child's ability to see him- or herself as valuable and good, and thus impedes the child's development of healthy self-respect. Whether the abuse occurred once or many times makes relatively little difference regarding the child's self-perception as bad, shameful, and worthless. It does appear that if the child was able to feel good about him- or herself prior to the onset of the abuse, he/she has a better chance for regaining this self-esteem later.

Given that the child victim was not respected by the abuser, and probably had little prior experience with demanding respect from others, the survivor will probably have great difficulty maintaining self-respect and the respect of others during adulthood.

The lack of self-respect and associated feelings of low self-worth and self-value may generate thoughts of self-injury in the survivor. Many survivors burn, cut, and bruise themselves in response to feelings of negative self-esteem, shame and guilt. For instance, when Ginny is criticized by her boss for sloppy work, Ginny's first and most compelling urge is to cut herself. Rather than hearing her boss say that her work needs improvement, Ginny hears that she is bad, and should be ashamed of herself. Her desire is to punish herself not only for her innate badness, but also for allowing someone else assume control and power over her. She is unable to maintain her self-respect and her self-perception as a good person, when faced with criticism.

Sometimes, this lack of self-respect can lead to even greater danger. The survivor who fails to maintain self-respect often does not demand respect from others. Survivors seeking intimate relationships may engage with disrespectful, abusive individuals because survivors may not require respect from their partners. James' story provides some insight:

My eldest brother abused me from the time I can remember, only, I didn't really think of it as abuse. I didn't really know what was OK and not OK in families. I saw my Mom and Dad go at each other when they were arguing, sometimes even throwing stuff. And I saw them kissing and hugging, sometimes right after those fights. I saw my sisters practicing kissing with one another and I watched my Dad hook my sister's bra up when she couldn't get it done. It just didn't seem to weird that my brother would come into the bathroom when I was showering and tell me to bend over, or for him to come into my bed at night and demand that I blow him. Later, I figured out that something really wrong had gone on in my house.

First of all, no matter how I tried to believe that my brother's abuse had no impact on me, I just couldn't think of myself as straight, not with what we had done. I led a gay lifestyle. It didn't end there. Every relationship I got into had the same feel to it: I would cook, clean and sexually serve my partner. I would submit unless told to act differently. I didn't really think I was capable of acting any other way. My brother taught me to be a servant, so I was.

One day, I sort of woke up to all this shit. I had gone off with this guy, and he was into some weird stuff. And when he handed me this leather outfit and dog collar, I put it on. He forced me on all fours and kept me there. I submitted and acted obediently for days, until one evening, he was preparing to have some friends over, and he wouldn't let me up. The guests finally arrived, and there I was in leather and chains, on all fours. That's when it hit me: "I'm not a dog! I'm a man, and I should be treated as a man!" Somehow, from somewhere deep inside me, was this little seed of self-respect, ready to be nourished and grown (it certainly took a hurricane for that seed to be uncovered!).

Unlike James, sometimes survivors are unable to develop that respect from within and may bind themselves to abusive relation-ships. Survivors are very familiar with abusive relationships and may feel more comfortable managing what is familiar to them. Unfortunately, some of these survivors die maintaining old patterns. Thousands and thousands of women die every year because they believe that, "Next time things will be different." They continue to return to these abusive relationships because they are afraid of the unfamiliar and unknown. They see themselves as emotionally and financially incapable of leaving the abusive relationships, so they go back, over and over, until that seed is uncovered, or until they die.

Survivors are extremely vulnerable to exploitation by others as a result of their lack of self-respect. In an abusive relationship, a survivor may not only be verbally, physically, and emotionally abused, but he/she may also be sexually abused again. Additionally, the abusive partner may abuse him/her financially, requiring the survivor to support the abusive partner. Often like the original perpetrator, the abusive partner may exploit the survivor by taking and distributing nude photographs of the survivor, by using the survivor as a prostitute or by engaging the survivor in the abuse of others, including children and animals.

Often, survivors become involved in a number of abusive relationships before they meet a healthy partner. During that first healthy relationship, the survivor is likely to act out, and to attempt to transform the relationship into another abusive situation, not because the survivor enjoys abuse, but because it is familiar. If these ideas ring true in your relationship, it is imperative that you resist your partner's "tests," in order for your partner to gain self-respect, and for the relationship to develop in a healthy fashion. In my work with survivors, I have seen many couples in which the survivor would bait his/her partner, goading the partner to respond to the survivor abusively, not only to prove that all partners are abusive, but to reset the relationship to a setting that is familiar to the survivor. And, as much as you may want to respond abusively after a number of these tests and trials, it is important that you refrain from becoming yet another abuser. The healthy partner can be one of the survivor's best allies in regaining and maintaining self-respect and self-esteem.

Exercise #29: "Tests I have encountered"

How does your partner test you?

What responses have you made so far?

What new alternatives have you learned from this book that you can try?

"What makes *you* so special?"

As we review the life of the survivor, we see again and again, pictures of shame, guilt and disdain. The perception that the survivor has of him- or herself as non-valuable, worthless, and bad pervades the survivor's life cycle and follows him/her everywhere. While other perceptions and ideas may be integrated with time, the original images may be quite durable.

Just as the abuser fails to respect the survivor's personal boundaries, he/she also fails to consider the survivor's needs or desires. Sexual abuse is about the satisfaction of the perpetrator's desires at the expense of another individual, without regard to consequence. From this abusive situation, especially if it is chronic, the survivor may learn that his or her needs are not important enough to consider. In the most abusive outcomes, survivors lend themselves to exploitation and physical abuse. In less abusive outcomes, survivors become co-dependent, and remain focused on the satisfaction of the needs of others in order to maintain their self-esteem. In the least abusive situation, the survivor martyrs him- or herself for the benefit of others, promoting an inherent sense of serenity. Yet, all of these consequences portray the survivor as at the mercy of someone else. The needs and desires of the survivor never enter the foreground.

In order for the survivor to develop independence and individuality, it is important that he/she recognize and act on his/her needs and desires. This consideration enables the survivor to feel empowered as an adult, reaching out to fill all of the needs that were previously denied. Unfortunately, when your partner begins working on the consideration of his/her own needs, you may experience this new egocentricism as overwhelming and isolating. You may even try to force your partner back into his/her old behavior. It is important that you work together to develop new, healthy habits and responses which allow each of you individuality, respect and power in the relationship. Each individual's needs and desires must be considered for the partnership to be successful.

In some cases, the survivor had access to other sources of support during the period of abuse. When the survivor has an ally, even if the abuse can not be terminated, the survivor may develop certain positive characteristics vicariously. While the survivor may be unable to recognize his/her own needs, he/she may be able to identify the needs of others, and may be able to respond with accuracy and kindness. When this is the case, the survivor may be able to relate to his/her partner with consideration and care. If the survivor has had very limited experience with consideration and has been unable to develop a consideration for self or others, the survivor may respond to his/her partner with indifference, taunting or sadism.

While it is important that your partner treat you with the respect and consideration you deserve, it may help to understand a little bit about why the survivor acts this way. The basic experience of the survivor is that of fear and shame. The survivor's shame prohibits him/her from talking about his/her problems with others, and the survivor's fear further isolates him/her. Originally, the survivor feared for his/her life, often maintaining the abuse to escape injury or death to self, sibling or parent. As deception became more imperative, the survivor feared discovery, and thus developed a mask or facade to hide the truth about the sexual abuse. Behind the mask lived a helpless, frightened child.

In addition to a deceptive facade, the survivor learned the abusive behaviors of the perpetrator and may have opted to take them on as his/her own. As the survivor becomes involved in intimate relationships, he/she continues to fear that his/her partner will discover the helplessness and vulnerability. To counteract, the survivor may use behaviors that he/she learned from his/her abuser and assume a dominant, insensitive role. In this case, the survivor may make demands of the partner without consideration of the partner's needs or desires. While it may seem as if you would be well aware if your partner were acting this way, consider Charlie's story:

> *She was so beautiful and charming, and she caught my eye in a heartbeat. I knew that I wanted to be with this woman, and I set out to meet her. We hit it off pretty well and began spending quite a lot of time together soon after we met at that party. She was worldly and well-traveled and we often talked about her life experiences. She liked to have me over to her place; I guess she liked to be on her own turf.*

> *I got to love the sound of her voice, as she dominated most conversations. I rationalized that she had more to talk about, because she'd done more and seen more. If I changed the subject, it would return to her, but I loved to hear about her life. She always chose where we would go, and she had such wonderful taste. She even ordered for us when we went out, because she was so much better at it than I was (she reminded me of that). She even like to shop for me, helping me to select just the right suit, because "I have much better taste than you!" She selected the place and time for our first sexual encounter, and it was better than I dreamed of. Then, she continued to schedule our sex life, at her convenience.*

*I loved her for her worldly charms and sophistica-
tion, and now that our relationship is over I can
safely say that I have never met a more domineer-
ing, narcissistic bitch in all of my life! She never
once considered my thoughts, feelings, desires or
needs, at any stage of our relationship, no matter
how basic or unsophisticated they might have
been.*

While some are raised with the ability to consider the needs,
thoughts and feelings that they have as well as those of others,
other individuals must be trained to do so. Survivors are trained
by their abusers to believe that their thoughts, feelings and
desires are unimportant, and barring input from other healthy
sources of support, survivors may not learn how to be
considerate of others. Survivors like others who do not learn
consideration during childhood, can learn to identify and respect
the thoughts, feelings, needs, and desires of their partners.

Exercise #30: "Giving and receiving empathy"

How much empathy are you capable of?
How about your partner?
How do you and your partner respond to each other's needs
and desires?

"Don't tell!"
If your partner was sexually abused by an individual outside
his/her family, he/she may have been able to develop a relatively
healthy communication style. The survivor still learned the vow
of silence from his/her perpetrator, but may have had allies to
assist him/her to speak out about other conflicts and issues. If
the survivor had a particularly healthy ally, it is possible that
the survivor even had early opportunities to disclose about the
abuse and begin to heal. If your partner was raised in an
incestuous family, his/her communication style is probably
based on the dysfunctional family motto, "Don't tell!" (In addition
to the threats of the perpetrator to remain silent).
Dysfunctional families, especially those in which members
are being sexually abused, focus their energies on maintaining
the illusion that things are OK, even if they must sacrifice one

of their members to do so. It is imperative that members uphold the facade by donning public masks so that others can not see their pain and distress. They must not speak to those in their surroundings, lest someone actually catch on. And, above all, these family members must not feel, because to do so would make the situation real and identifiable.

If a member cannot follow the guidelines, no matter how strong the demands by the rest of the family, that member may be sacrificed or excluded. Frequently, in incestuous families, when a survivor confronts his/her family about the abuse, the survivor is not believed, even when the supportive evidence is strong. In order for the family to continue functioning in its dysfunctional pattern, it is necessary for that family to cut its losses, supporting only those who follow the rules of ignorance and silence. Logistically, this may mean that the survivor is allowed to remain in the family but is shunned by the other members, or that the survivor may be barred from family interactions. Either way, the survivor ends up emotionally, physically, and socially isolated.

In their isolation, incest survivors rarely learn how to communicate openly with others. Not only does the family teach them that "Silence is Golden," but they are often confused further by their abusers. During the abuse, the perpetrator may have told the survivor, "I love you," then caused intense physical and emotional pain. The sensory mismatch between the verbal behavior ("I love you") and the non-verbal behavior (sexually forcing and hurting the child) causes the child to become confused. Most people pay greater attention to the non-verbal information they receive, but will try to make sense of any additional information available. The incest survivor knows that he/she has been physically invaded and hurt, but wants to believe what the perpetrator has said. In future intimate relationships, these survivors will have trouble believing what they hear, especially if it varies from what they see or experience.

If we consider the "Don't tell!" rule, and the sensory mismatches provided by perpetrators and other family members (like non-protective parents or siblings who also profess their love and concern), it seems realistic that survivors often find communication with others difficult and strained. It is unlikely that anyone living in a family with the "Don't tell!" rule in place is going to communicate assertively, as this would require the individual to first feel, then disclose to others. Given the climate of incestuous (and most dysfunctional) families, it is more likely that survivors will learn a more passive or aggressive communication style.

Survivors who withdraw into the isolation generated by the sexual abuse often develop a passive way of coping with the world in general. They step out of conflict situations, retreat when arguments heat up, shut down when emotions are high, and hide when they feel overwhelmed. When confronted, they are likely to submit rather than face the possible consequences for opposition or rebellion. If the survivor experiences anger, resentment or disappointment, and wishes to express it, he/she will most likely do so with a passive/aggressive style.

Recall John and Delia in the last chapter. When Delia was angry at John for failing to meet her hidden expectations, Delia subtly destroyed John's plans for a relaxing evening at home. In this way, she was able to behave vengefully, without taking the responsibility for her feelings nor expressing them to John.

Another common style of communication for survivors, aggression, was mentioned briefly in the last section. Sometimes, survivors who endure especially harsh sexual abuse, or who experience overwhelming feelings of helplessness and isolation will form a trauma bond or identify with their abuser(s) in order to feel that they are in greater control. In addition to empathizing with their abusers, survivors may develop behaviors and communication styles similar to those of their abusers. For example, a large percentage of boys who endure physical or sexual abuse by their fathers or who witness abuse of their mothers by their fathers, end up abusing the women in their lives. While they may hate themselves for repeating the cycle, they behave as they have been taught to behave by their fathers, in the only fashion that would have been safe should their fathers have witnessed. Such behavior is based on the dominant, macho He-Man stereotype that has been maintained for many generations of men, barred from feeling and expressing their sensitivity and gentleness.

Men aren't the only survivors who may identify with their abusers. Patty Hearst is a famous example of a female kidnapping survivor who identified with her abductors in order to remain alive and mentally intact. While this coping strategy facilitated her survival, she later replaced it with healthier, less primitive coping strategies. Subsequent to her release and debriefing, she married her bodyguard. Many less celebrated women have also identified with their abusers in order to cope with abuse. Some have chosen to facilitate abuse of others, and some have become perpetrators themselves. These survivors communicate to the world what they know, in the only way they know how. In order to really hear what these survivors are saying, you may have to pay close attention to how they are saying it. For more information on "trauma bonding" see the works of Jan Hindman.

Assertive communication is a skill, and anyone can learn to speak to others in a clear, respectful, yet honest fashion. Survivors are no exception: while they often emerge from families enmeshed in silence, survivors can move into the light and learn to communicate their thoughts, feelings, needs and desires to their families, friends, colleagues and lovers.

Exercise #31: "How my partner and I communicate"

What is your communication style?
Does it change with mood or situation?
How about your partner's?
How do you promote or inhibit assertive communication?

"How can you really know how I feel?"

As a partner and ally to the survivor, you must accept this one thing: you will never really know how the survivor feels. Even if you, too, are a survivor, it is unlikely that your abuse situations were identical, and though you may share similar thoughts and feelings, you can't ever really know what it was like for your partner. That doesn't mean that you can't learn to empathize and support the survivor. You can learn to understand more about the survivor by trying to place yourself in his/her shoes and walking around for a bit. You can read other books like this one, and listen to more stories of survivors in order to really get acquainted with the world of the survivor, but you're never really going to know.

The individual who survives sexual abuse is isolated by the physical and emotional events which occur. There is a certain sadness and grief that survivors experience as they are stripped of their innocent and playful childhood bodies, lives, fantasies and games. Survivors are often overwhelmed by the sadness associated with their isolation and loneliness. They can not really engage with others because of THE SECRET. They do not really feel playful after THE SECRET has begun. They hide in order to soothe their ragged bodies, lying down or crouching in order to allow their bodies to heal. Survivors may not have been able to move quickly enough or flexibly enough to play with other children, depending on the kind and intensity of the abuse they endured. They can not really bond because THE SECRET always gets in the way. Some survivors withdraw and grieve and try to hide from their perpetrators, and other survivors try to go on, as if nothing has happened, until later, usually in late adolescence or young adulthood, when they can no longer hold the grief at bay. And then, the survivor is consumed, often unaware of the source of his/her grief. And within this grief and sadness is the inability to connect with others and to share the horrible SECRET. It is this lack of connection that the survivor references when he/she says, "How can you really know how I feel?" Because, as his/her partner, you can't know, as no one in the survivor's surroundings could, because the survivor was isolated, left alone to deal with the abuse and the grief.

The second feeling associated with this lack of understanding by others is rage. Often when the survivor asks, "How can you really know how I feel?" there is a silent accusation attached to the question. The survivor was indeed isolated during and after the abuse, without a soul to assist and protect him/her. You can never really know how the survivor feels because you weren't there (for the survivor). You, as the most intimate connection the survivor now has, may become the representative of all those who were not there to protect the survivor from the abuse. While you are not to blame for the abuse that he/she endured, he/she may symbolically use you in order to confront those who did not protect him/her in the past. In this case, it is imperative that you are supportive and objective, otherwise, you are likely to become defensive, especially if the survivor uses an accusatory tone with you! The survivor may be comforted by statements such as, "I'm sorry I wasn't there to protect you." "I'm angry that those people who were there didn't protect you," or "I'm trying to understand but it's hard because I wasn't there. Help me understand you better now."

As your partner learns to trust you, through repeated testing, he/she may become more honest and allow him- or herself to be more vulnerable with you. In order to help your partner become comfortable with this increased, "safe" vulnerability, it is important that you recognize the risk that the survivor makes in order to share with you in this way. As it will allow for greater intimacy in your relationship, it is imperative that you nurture each effort that the survivor makes to open up and disclose about him- or herself. (In the next chapter, you will find some guidelines for responding to disclosures of abuse). As you learn to communicate more honestly with one another, you will both be surprised at how much you can understand about one another!

Exercise #32: "Connecting"

How are you and your partner able to connect?

When are those connections inhibited?

How do you respond when your partner has trouble connecting?

"How soon will I be betrayed?"

For the survivor, it is often not a question of whether or not he/she will be betrayed in the future, but rather, when the betrayal will occur. Since the onset of the abuse, and possibly even prior to the abuse, it is likely that the survivor has been unable to trust him- or herself, or anyone else. Because the survivor may feel that he/she cannot even trust his/her own instincts, body, and mind, it may seem impossible to develop trust with anyone else, even within the context of an intimate relationship.

With the onset of the abuse, the survivor begins to question his/her basic instincts and ideas about him- or herself and about those in his/her environment. Since most abuse is committed by an individual that the survivor knows and with whom he/she has frequent contact, the survivor has often become trusting of the potential perpetrator. The survivor may perceive the potential perpetrator as an important, reliable, powerful friend and mentor. And, when this individual violates the personal and relational boundaries set by the child, this would-be friend and mentor becomes a cruel abuser, destroying the child's sense of security and trust in those in the world around him/her.

Often more significantly, the perpetration demolishes the survivor's ability to trust him- or herself and the basic instincts that the survivor has held about people. In this case, the survivor may ask him- or herself repeatedly, "How could I have been so trusting? Why couldn't I see that this person was going to hurt me?" The survivor may lose faith in his/her ability to judge the intentions and sincerity of others, and may stop trusting completely.

Additionally, if the survivor's body responded to the abuse (e.g. if you stroke a male's penis, it will become erect), the survivor may feel that his/her own body has betrayed him/her. The survivor is unable to rely on the most basic entity available to him/her for support.

Given the effects which sexual abuse has on the survivor's ability to trust him- or herself and others, it may be difficult for the partner to become intimate with the survivor. The development of trust in an intimate relationship with a survivor is probably second only to the struggle for control within that relationship.

For the survivor to begin to develop trust with others, he/she must first begin this work at the core: the survivor must learn once again to trust his/her body and mind, and to tune back into the basic instincts and intuitions that are often turned off or tuned out following the onset of abuse. Forgiving the body is probably the easier of these two tasks, as the survivor can learn about the body's basic "hardwiring" and the effects which manual stimulation has on every human body. While this task may not be easy, the retraining is logical, and may thus be more acceptable to the survivor. The end result of learning more about the body and how it works, is that the survivor gets his/her body back, and can begin to regain the private sexuality lost with the first perpetration.

Learning to trust his/her instincts and intuitions may be even harder for the survivor. His/her memory holds evidence that those instincts were somehow wrong in the past, and it is often difficult for the survivor to accept that lying and manipulating is the perpetrator's forte. As the survivor begins to learn more about the phenomena of sexual abuse, and about how perpetrators initiate and maintain the abuse of children and adolescents, the trust of instincts is slowly regained. Survivors may need constant reassurance and frequent reminders to trust their inner "parenting" voice. It is important that the survivor learn to differentiate between intuition and the voice of the frightened inner child, who may demand that the survivor protect and control himself/herself even when the circumstances do not require this. Derek's story clarifies this:

I really had a hard time with that stuff when I was in graduate school. I was alone and didn't know anyone and really needed some guidance. I wanted to learn, so that I could do well, get ahead, and feel successful and proud of myself, but it was really hard to know the ins and outs of the system during that first year. When Professor Adams took a liking to me, and started to help me wade through the material, one part of me was so happy and grateful. That part felt like I'd hit the Mother Lode, and finally had the mentor I'd been searching for. I tried to hold on to the voice, and to read it as a good instinct about him, but damn it if way down deep there wasn't this scared little boy piping up to say, "Get away! Get out of there! He's going to hurt you! He can't be trusted. No man can! You'll see, he's going to be just like Dad was."

My therapist spent a lot of time helping me to soothe that little boy, and be a much better parent to that part of myself than anyone else had ever been. Usually, if that young part of me could be soothed and calmed, then my other, positive instincts were on target. When that little boy was adamant, I listened and followed his lead.

Once the survivor can learn to trust him- or herself, it is possible for the survivor to begin to test, and ultimately trust others. As was suggested in the last section, the survivor must learn to cope with the sadness and rage associated with the abuse, in order to perceive the partner realistically as an ally rather than as another potential perpetrator. In addition to the therapeutic work that the survivor does on his/her own, the partner must actively work to explore his or her own trustworthiness, and ability to trust the survivor. If both partners continue to learn and grow, and to support one another in this process, lovers and survivors can strengthen the bond between them and build trust that can allow them greater freedom within the relationship to be vulnerable and honest.

Exercise #33: "Inner children, inner voices"

How connected are you to your own "inner voice" and intuition? Consider the last time that you were in a tight spot or scary situation: What did you tell yourself? What messages did you attend to? Why?

"How could I possibly let you in?"

Unfortunately for the partnership, survivors often associate vulnerability with the fear of abuse and death. To the survivor, to be vulnerable means to be small, helpless, and intimidated. The adult survivor usually has difficulty maintaining his/her adult identity when he/she feels vulnerable, making vulnerability a negatively-valued position. In order for individuals to feel close to one another, each must make an effort to be vulnerable and open to the impact and the essence of the other. This relational paradox is one of the most common struggles between lovers and survivors.

For the survivor, the opening or the exposure of his/her true self historically resulted in physical, emotional and psychological abuse and confusion. In incestuous families, the child remained open to the impact of his/her parents, siblings and relatives because these were the very people that the child was supposed to be able to trust and after whom he/she could model him- or herself. When family members violate that trust, the child survivor is caught off-guard and is often left feeling completely isolated and unsupported. The experience of vulnerability in the incestuous family leaves the survivor in utter despair and without resources with which to cope. Given the result, it is unlikely that the survivor will open him- or herself to similar torment again. The survivor will seek a position of power, and will attempt to control the flow of information, so that the survivor is always in the driver's seat and avoids experiencing the terror of vulnerability. Few relationships can function in a healthy way if one individual is always controlling and the other is always submitting or concurring. When the survivor enters a love relationship, he/she struggles with the archaic issues of the past, in order to move forward into intimacy with his/her partner.

Generally, the survivor will test his/her partner repeatedly to determine whether the partner is trustworthy, and whether or not the partner will take advantage of the survivor. For instance, in the initial stages of the relationship, survivors often provoke and encourage their partners to take advantage of them sexually. If the partner does the survivor concludes that the partner is another perpetrator and likely moves on. If the partner refuses to exploit the survivor's sexual vulnerability, the survivor will either provoke the partner further (trying to determine the extent of the partner's good will) or will accept the partner as a healthy partner and will cease the testing.

Should the partner pass all of the survivor's "tests," the survivor may be willing to attempt some form of vulnerability, perhaps sharing personal thoughts or aspirations, or even details about the abuse. While these actions may appear to be basic to the partner, to the survivor, the process may feel like life-threatening exposure. Given that, it is important that the partner treat the disclosures and attempts at vulnerability as special and valuable. The more comfortable the survivor becomes with sharing information, the more likely he/she is to open herself further to impact by his/her partner. As intimacy increases between the partners, the less the survivor will associate vulnerability with feelings of helplessness and the fear of abuse and death.

Exercise #34: "Managing vulnerability"

How do you accept your own vulnerability? Make a list of the things that you do to avoid or accept feeling vulnerable, especially when interacting with others.

"You want me to do WHAT?"

Even if the partners are able to achieve the healthy communication and response style of an intimate relationship, at some point, the couple must recognize their mutual sexuality. As stated previously, for the couple to engage in mutual sexual interaction, there must be consent, equality, respect, trust, safety and compatibility. If any of these factors is missing, there is danger that one partner will be abused or exploited.

Given the survivor's historical experience, it is imperative that all sexual interactions be mutually consenting. If there is a question, or if it seems as if consent has been implied, CHECK WITH YOUR PARTNER! Make certain that your desires are mutual before advancing sexually.

Equality is important for the same reason. Should one partner be in control of the sexual situation, the other partner may feel passive, helpless, or exploited. You may find that the survivor demands greater control during sexual interaction. If this is mutually acceptable, then allow the survivor the freedom to control the situation so that he/she can feel safe to interact with you.

Respect between partners is important in any situation but respect between sexual partners is imperative. The desires and needs of each partner must be considered and responded to, even if that means separating shortly before climax! When one partner needs more space, or a break from the sexual interaction, it is important that his/her partner treats the request with respect. Whether and when sexual interaction resumes is up to both partners.

Sexual interaction should not occur if both partners do not trust one another and feel safe. Because sex requires the individual to be in the most vulnerable position, he/she must feel safe in the setting and with his/her partner in order to relax and enjoy him- or herself. When survivors engage in sex with individuals that they do not trust or with whom they do not feel safe, it recreates the abusive situation, and endangers the survivor's healing and emotional health. Danger may arise in the form of an abusive partner or may be reflected in flashbacks of past abuse. In the latter situation, the survivor may experience the current situation as abuse from the past, likely unaware of his/her current surroundings or partner, and attending only to the memory of the past, as if it were occurring in the present.

In addition to these basic components for mutual sexual interaction, partners need to be compatible in a number of ways. For instance, the sexual preferences of the couple must be in concert. While it may seem as if sexual preference would be obvious, occasionally, that is not the case. The formation of a sexual identity is often a difficult task for the survivor, and he/she may develop an identity subsequent to the abuse which is different from the identity he/she had maintained prior to the abuse. For example, there are those survivors who identify themselves as heterosexual prior to and following the abuse. There are other female survivors who identify themselves as heterosexual prior to the abuse, but identify themselves as lesbian following the abuse. While some women choose the lesbian lifestyle in response to abuse by men, other survivors claim to have been unaware of their lesbian identities until after the abuse. Finally, other females are aware of their homosexual identities prior to the abuse and do not alter these identities no matter what the gender of the perpetrator is. Maltz and Holman (1987) refer to the different identities as "lesbian-born" versus "lesbian-bred."

Similarly, some male survivors have been unable to identify their homosexual identities until after the abuse ("gay-born"), while other male survivors learn to lead homosexual lifestyles following abuse by men, because they believe that the homosexual interaction has transformed them into homosexuals ("gay-bred"). Other males become hyper-sexual with women in order to constantly assert their heterosexual masculinity (this may lead to various forms of sexual addiction). Finally, while some survivors are aware of their bisexuality prior to the abuse, others only recognize their bisexual identities after the abuse ("bisexual-born"). Those survivors who are unable to choose a sexual identity and simply interact with every acceptable partner might be referred to as "bisexual-bred."

In addition to compatible sexual preferences, each partner's level of sexual emergence must mesh with the other's. As noted in other chapters, survivors often run to the extremes in terms of sexual behavior: either they are sexually withdrawn and resistant or they are promiscuous and non-discerning. Sexual emergence appears to be relative to the degree to which the survivor has healed his/her sexuality. For instance, the sexual abuse survivor who has yet to face her issues may repeatedly enter relationships which are sexualized and which have little other substance, as she repeats the behaviors with which she has been made familiar due to her chronic abuse. The promiscuity of this survivor is consistent with her abusive training.

On the other hand, the abuse survivor who has spent some time working through abuse issues may be much more relaxed in his/her sexuality, developing mutual sexual interaction in relationships when the couple has developed a trusting, intimate bond that will withstand the intensity of sexual passion.

Finally, it is important that the partners agree on mutual sexual interests and boundaries. As we saw in Chapter 5, the kinds of sexual interactions desired by partners may not always be compatible. While most survivors can heal their sexuality to include any behaviors and situations they wish, such healing

142 • S. Yvette de Beixedon, Ph.D.

and integration takes time. As a partner, it is important to recognize that the process may take a great deal of time and energy from both members of the couple.

Additionally, survivors may have a number of limitations to their sexuality. What those limitations are depends on the survivor and his/her experience of abuse. For instance, while many female survivors find it extremely uncomfortable to have their partner enter them from behind, other survivors are much more comfortable with this position. If a survivor has been raped in the rear entry position or has been sodomized, this position of vulnerability is likely to be the last sexual frontier that he/she will confront.

While limitations to sexuality are rarely permanent if the survivor and his/her partner agree to work on these obstacles separately and together, they certainly present stressors in the relationship that might not otherwise be there. While sexuality is often a form of play and comfort for some couples, survivors and their lovers may find sexual interaction to be confusing, challenging and frustrating. It is important that the couple who is working toward more satisfying sexual interaction, identify at least one sexual behavior that is safe, non-threatening, and enjoyable. As the survivor accomplishes greater and greater sexual healing, the couple may discover more forms of sexual interaction which they can enjoy.

Exercise #35: "Sharing intimacy"

Find a quiet place, free of distractions and intrusions and sit down with your partner. Each of you take pen and paper to make a list of the intimate activities that you can do without fear, shame or rage. When your lists are complete, take turns sharing these with one another. Then, order the list from least challenging to most challenging. Select activities that are fairly easy to begin experimenting with in your relationship. When you are ready, move on to activities that are harder!

"How can I give to myself what I give to others?"

Individuals who have been sexually abused may have felt unable to identify or empathize with others. They may have experienced so much isolation and rage within their abusive environments that they felt unable to connect with others who had similar feelings. They may also have feared empathy, lest they excuse their perpetrators for having abused them, invalidating their very experience. More often, survivors are most sensitive to the pain of others and empathize deeply. They often make excellent counselors and therapists, doctors and customer service representatives. Every time the survivor is able to experience that other person's pain, rage, and guilt, the survivor gets to experience and release just a bit of his/her own pain. As the survivor empathizes and attends to that other person's feelings, the survivor gets some vicarious comfort and empathy. Until the survivor can meet his/her needs for empathy directly, the painful, intense feelings associated with the abuse will remain suppressed below the surface.

In order for the survivor to accept empathy from others, he/she needs to learn how to empathize with the abused part of him- or herself (or the "inner child"). Empathy for the self requires that the survivor give up the total control that he/she might otherwise maintain. When the controlled facade is rolled back, the survivor must be willing to face the feelings of overwhelming helplessness, rage, resentment, and fear. And when the survivor is able to experience those feelings and survive the reality of the abuse, he/she can let go of the inner child so that it can be integrated into the total personality.

Most survivors find that in order to integrate the abused part (which has been disconnected from the "adult self" for so long), they must "re-parent" the inner child. When the abused part begins to demand safety and protection when this is not called for, the survivor can talk to that part of him- or herself, soothing the inner child, and calming that young part with a healthy parenting voice. The only trouble with this process is that if the survivor was abused by one or both parents, or experienced the parents as non-protective or insensitive caretakers, the survivor may not have learned a healthy "parenting voice." In this case, the survivor must learn to re-parent from role models in his/her surroundings (e.g. from her partner's family, friends, healthy relatives, TV, books, media or movies). As the survivor is able to better and better empathize with, forgive, and comfort the abused part of him or her, an increasing percentage of the old self is integrated. This process then enables the survivor to receive empathy and comfort from others, especially from his/her partner.

Exercise #36: "Developing your parenting voice"

Find a quiet place to sit where you will not be distracted for at least a half-hour. Now visualize yourself in a frightening or nerve-wracking situation. Now let your inner voice calm and soothe you. Open your eyes, and make a list of the phrases that would comprise your "parenting voice."

"What do you mean it wasn't my fault?"

Just as the survivor must learn to empathize with that abused part of him- or herself before the survivor can comfortably receive empathy and comfort from others, the survivor must also identify and let go of the shame and guilt associated with the abuse, in order to feel compassion from self and others. Since the survivor may have assumed a sense of guilt in order to experience some sense of control over the abuse, it may be difficult for the survivor to let go of the old coping strategy.

For the survivor to experience compassion for himself or herself, it will be necessary for him/her to forgive the abused inner child for being vulnerable to the perpetrator. The survivor must recognize that he/she was not to blame in order to release his/her sense of shame and guilt. As the survivor meets and shares with other survivors, he/she will begin to differentiate between healthy shame (i.e. that prohibits us as adults from pulling our clothes off in public) and unhealthy shame (which maintains the silence of the abuse). As shame is reduced, the compassion for self increases, and the survivor can begin to appreciate all of the positive qualities that he/she has, some even as a result of his/her abuse and subsequent survival.

In order for the survivor to let go of old, unhealthy, shame-maintaining habits, he/she will need the support of others to do so. As a partner, it will be important to be sensitive to those situations in which your partner is likely to experience shame and guilt, and support him/her through those times, offering frequent validation and reinforcement. When your partner attempts to take the responsibility for events that are beyond his/her control, help him/her recognize that he/she is not responsible, and as uncomfortable as it may be to allow someone else to take control of those events, it is healthier for him/her to remain true to himself or herself. As much compassion as you offer to the survivor, you merit as much compassion in return. Just because your partner has been sexually abused does not mean that he/she can use you as a caretaker without considering your needs as well. When the survivor is in therapy and/or working through abuse issues, he/she may be more self-absorbed than normal and may not be as sensitive to your needs and desires as you would like him/her to be. If this is the case, confront the survivor lovingly and assert your needs and feelings. Be compassionate to one another.

Exercise #37: "Responses to shame"

In what situations do you feel shamed?

How do you need others to respond to you in those situations?

If your partner is willing, review some of the situations in which he/she feels shamed.

How can you help your partner to let go of shame?

"What? We can have fun?"

Survivors are often ruled by their inner children, and their rationales for events and practices frequently have the magical quality of the child's thought processes. For example, many survivors enjoyed pleasant childhood until being abused, and may have associated the experience of pleasure or happiness with impending doom. In this way, survivors are often afraid to have fun, lest they "be punished" for letting things get too good. The logic makes sense to the child, even though it may be farfetched to the mature adult!

Similarly, it is often the case that survivors who were raised in physically, emotionally and sexually abusive homes were beaten or punished for positive, lively, or joyful behavior. For example, one young child who was raised in a sexually abusive and extremely religious home returned from school, quite proud of his outstanding report card. His mother, who believed that pride was sacrilegious, stripped him, chained him to a wall, and repeatedly whipped his genitalia until he passed out. Survivors who were punished or demeaned for being positive or having fun are not likely to play of their own accord.

Survivors who assume some responsibility for the abuse may believe that they do not deserve to have interests or hobbies which could bring them pleasure. Even if the survivor felt worthy of play, abusive parents or teachers may have restricted the survivor.

In any case, it is often true that survivors do not develop interests and remain isolated and withdrawn.

The absence of play creates at least two problems: first, play is an essential part of human existence, providing nourishment for the body and spirit. Therefore, when survivors do not give themselves the opportunity for play, they continue to deplete their energies without replenishing the supply. Secondly, play often reflects our interests and desires. When the survivor does not play, he/she misses the opportunity for interacting with others who enjoy the same interests. When play is restricted, not only does the survivor continue to deplete his/her vital energy, but he/she also remains isolated and without the support he/she so greatly needs.

In order for the survivor to truly heal, and develop a self that is healthy and able to interact fully with others, it is imperative that he/she learn to play. As it is often difficult for the survivor to generate ideas for play by him- or herself (due to lack of experience or shame associated with play), I highly encourage partners to help their survivors play. And as play between two people can create deeply emotional and intense bonds, it can bring the couple closer together, while allowing each to take care of his/her own needs for replenishment and release.

Exercise #38: "Having fun!"

With your partner, make a list of all the playful activities you can do, separately and together, no matter how simple or "childish" they may seem. Once your list is completed, randomly select an activity from your list, and go have fun!

Chapter 7
Being a Partner

The chapters that have preceded this one have informed you about child and adolescent sexual abuse and its impacts on the survivor's physical, emotional and psychological health, and have identified some of the impacts that sexual abuse has on your ability to intimately interact with one another. The changes, modifications and limitations to the survivor have been addressed and explained, but what about your experience? So far, some of the obstacles that you face have been identified, but not much has been said about the emotional upheaval that you may experience as a result of your relationship with the survivor. As this text is meant to assist you in your personal and relational challenges with the survivor, let's address now some of the unique experiences you may have.

Most therapists and researchers would agree that when an individual becomes involved with a survivor of sexual abuse, he/she also becomes a victim "by association or attachment." Some call partners "co-survivors" or "pro-survivors," but whatever the term, you can be sure that the individual who becomes involved with a survivor experiences many thoughts and feelings similar to those of the survivor, as well as a host of other intense feelings. Unfortunately, while the survivor is provided with various forms of support and resources during his/her healing process, the partner may not receive the same kind of treatment or compassion from others (maybe not even from the survivor).

Just as survivors experience physical, emotional, psychological, behavioral, and social impacts of sexual abuse, partners encounter similar effects when the survivor initially discloses about his/her abuse, and often as you participate in the healing process. Many of the reactions that partners may have are negative and have the potential to worsen the relationship between lover and survivor. For this reason, it is imperative that both parties take active roles in understanding the sexual abuse and its effects. This dual participation will ensure that control of the relationship remains between the two of you. Some of the changes and impacts which follow the disclosure of sexual abuse and must be managed by both partner and survivor are outlined below.

Physical Impacts for the Partner

While you may not have to cope with the physical consequences of having been sexually abused (unless you are also a survivor), you may experience a number of physical symptoms and changes subsequent to the survivor's initial disclosure. Most individuals go into shock while listening to the survivor's story, especially if the details are especially gruesome or if the partner is fond of the perpetrator. Jack relates some of his experience below:

> After Glynnis and I were married, I got to know her older brother pretty well. We'd hang out, go to the ball game together, you know, just pal around. I really enjoyed his company, and Glynnis never really minded if I was out with Mark. After Mark wrecked his car, things changed. Mark broke some bones and was laid up in the hospital, and after Glyn saw him, she started freaking out. I guess that's when she popped her first memory of the abuse.

> We didn't really know what was happening to Glynnis, so I took her to see a counselor. Within only a few visits, Glynnis had recover-ed a lot of her memories, and that's when she asked me to come to therapy with her. We sat there together, and I didn't know what was coming next, thinking crazy thoughts like, "She's going to leave me!", "She's found someone else!" And then, the therapist helped her tell me what Mark had done to her as a kid. It was so bad that she blocked it all out, until she saw him there, helpless, and childlike in that hospital. I guess it reminded her of when he was young.

> Anyway, when they told me, I remember shaking my head and saying, "Not Mark! Not the guy I hang out with! He could never do anything like that to you! He's so keen on you..." And, then I looked up at her, and I saw her face streaming with tears and I knew that she'd never lie about something like this, and I thought, "Oh, my God, what's

happening? How could this be?" I hugged her hard, and I told her that I believed her and that I'd stand by her, whatever she wanted I'd do. But on the inside, my heart was beating a mile a minute, my thoughts were racing, I felt like throwing up, and my head was pounding so hard, I thought it was going to explode. After the session, we just sat in the car, staring out the window, totally dazed and confused, unable to think clearly enough to drive.

Jack's experience is a fairly common one. Often the couple has been together for some time, when something traumatic occurs which triggers the survivor's memory, and the couple together must manage the newly discovered trauma and its impacts. Alternatively, the survivor may enter the relationship, aware of his/her past history, and may make an intimate disclosure to the partner. In any case, the story generally impacts the partner immediately in a variety of ways. The shock described by Jack is often the first physical impact. Initial disclosure may leave the partner with the following physical symptoms:

- headache or migraine
- tightness in the jaw and face
- dry mouth
- tears
- tightness or "clutching" in the throat ("lump in the throat")
- sore shoulder and neck muscles
- tight fists
- increased blood pressure
- heart pounding
- cold sweats
- body shakes
- nausea
- weak knees
- temporary numbness in the hands and feet
- low back pain

While most of these physical symptoms recede with time, long-term partners occasionally find that a host of physical symptoms will remain. The most common physical complaints of partners include headaches or migraines, tightness in the throat, low back pain, and recurrent visual images of the abuse (that the partner has created in response to the survivor's disclosure). While it is less common, occasionally partners will experience sympathetic or vicarious physical pain, in the areas in which the survivor was abused. This experience is generally intense and fleeting, and usually occurs as the survivor is relating his/her past experiences of abuse.

Exercise #39: "Recognizing physical symptoms"

Take a few moments to relax and think. Consider how you've been feeling physically since your partner told you about the sexual abuse. What kinds of changes in your physical functioning have you noticed? Take five minutes to jot down the symptoms you recognize in yourself since beginning to deal with these issues.

In addition to the physical symptoms that you may be enduring, partners often experience a change in their sexuality as they attempt to cope with the disclosure. For a short period following the disclosure, it is normal for the partner to experience some loss of sexual desire, decreased arousal, and even sexual dysfunction or impotence. As the couple works together to learn more about the healing process and the impacts of sexual abuse, these initial physical responses may diminish for the partner.

If the survivor is just beginning to explore his/her issues, it is likely that he/she will avoid his/her sexuality and may completely shun sexual contact for a period of time. Should you make sexual advances toward your partner, you may be met by excuses to avoid sex, feelings of fear, and even disgust, even if you have enjoyed a healthy sexual relationship with your partner prior to the disclosure. While you may experience this rejection as an attack of your positive sexuality, it is important to recognize the survivor's limited ability to differentiate between sexuality and sexual abuse. As the survivor learns to better differentiate between the two, he/she will learn to accept not only his/her own sexuality, but will also learn to accept and affirm your sexuality as well.

Even during this potentially troublesome period, intimacy will continue to be important for the maintenance of the relationship, and it is important for the two of you to come to an agreement about the kind of sexual relationship you will have (even if this means that you hold hands in order to feel close rather than having intercourse while the survivor works through these issues).

Exercise #40: "Recognizing impacts to your sexual relationship"

If you have not done so already, take some time to sit down with your partner to discuss the impacts that disclosure and exploration of the sexual abuse has had on your sexual relationship. Let your partner identify any new positive or negative responses that he or she has noticed. Then, try to identify any changes that you have recognized in yourself. When you feel like you understand one another's experience, come to an agreement about the activities with which you can experiment to maintain intimacy. Make a list and keep it where you can both review and consult it as often as you like.

Partners may find relief from their somatic complaints when they are able to express their feelings about the disclosure and its impacts on the relationship, as emotions indisputably affect the body and its functioning. When an individual has entered a relationship with a survivor, or when memories of abuse have been disclosed, it is often helpful for the partner to receive counseling and support for his/her response to the disclosure.

Emotional Effects

In addition to the physical symptoms that you may endure, partners experience a number of different emotions in response to disclosure of sexual abuse. Some of the emotions that you may be experiencing closely resemble those experienced by the survivor both during and after the abuse. Emotions experienced by partners include but are not limited to:

- shock
- disbelief
- confusion
- resentment
- disappointment
- anger, rage

- frustration
- blame
- shame, embarrassment
- disgust
- sadness
- helplessness
- despair
- hopelessness

Many of these emotions were apparent in Jack's response to Glynnis' news, though other emotions may arise subsequent to the initial disclosure. Most partners experience the shock, confusion, and disbelief noted by Jack. Some partners are unable to tolerate the other emotions and remain emotionally neutral or blank following the disclosure. More commonly, partners cry and shout, terribly sad for what the survivor has experienced and enraged that another human being could so abuse a child.

Some partners uphold their commitment to the relationship with the survivor and participate actively in the healing process. These partners are likely to be honest about their own feelings about the disclosure and the abuse. If the couple has been together for some time before the survivor discloses, the partner will likely feel resentful and disappointed in the survivor. The partner may interpret the survivor's delay in disclosing the abuse as limited trust in the partner, and may be disappointed that the survivor did not open up sooner. These partners may experience negative emotional reactions to the disclosure, but are likely to support their abused partners and will allow the "blame" to rest with the perpetrator.

Other partners may not feel comfortable sharing their emotional reactions with the survivor, and may keep their feelings hidden or suppressed. Generally, this suppression of emotions results in resentment toward the survivor and an emotional explosion somewhere down the line. If the resentment is great enough, the partner may even attempt to blame the survivor for the conflicts which arise within the relationship, or even for the original abuse. While I believe that supportive therapy can greatly assist all those who interact with abuse survivors, therapy is especially important for those partners who are unable to empathize with their abused partners. Not so infrequently, these partners are also survivors of physical or sexual abuse.

Some partners are embarrassed about the subject of sexual abuse and may inhibit any discussion that the survivor initiates. These partners are likely to identify with the survivor's sense of shame about the abuse. It is important that the partner not increase the level of shame experienced by the survivor as a result of his/her own discomfort with the subject. If your partner has tried to speak with you about his/her abuse, and you have felt too uncomfortable to hear his/her story, it is important that you take responsibility for your feelings. If you cannot bear to participate in the survivor's healing, let him/her know that you care, but are not able to cope with the disclosure. Encourage the survivor to talk and share with supportive friends and relatives, and to use a professional listener (counselor). Additionally, offer your support to the survivor in different ways.

Exercise #41: "Emotional responses to disclosure of sexual abuse"

Has your partner disclosed a history of sexual abuse to you? If so, how did you feel when you heard his or her story? Take ten minutes, and try to list as many of your emotional reactions to your partner's disclosure as you can.

Individuals who are reexperiencing and integrating abuse experiences often feel isolated, ashamed, frightened, and stressed. They generally experience a wide range of physical, emotional and psychological changes as they heal, and may need assistance in more than one area. If you are unable to share your partner's efforts to "break the silence," then you can offer support in other ways: when the survivor's body is tense and aching, you can offer to rub his/her arms, shoulders or feet. If the survivor feels unsafe when memories are returning, develop a ritual with your partner: help the survivor lock doors that are unlocked, close windows that are open and find special, safe objects or places that offer a sense of security to the survivor. When the survivor is employing enormous amounts of energy to heal and regroup, offer to clean the house, cook a meal, or shop for the survivor, or offer to take the survivor to a safe, recuperative place that has no association to the abuse (take a break for fun!). You don't have to hear the story if you feel that you can't, but that doesn't mean you can't help the survivor heal in other important ways.

Finally, it is vital that you, as a partner, understand and accept that healing from sexual abuse takes a lifetime. The physical, emotional, and psychological scars are indelible and cannot ever be removed. And, as the trauma impacts the very being of the survivor, it is important that those scars remain and that memories be integrated, in order for the survivor to be reminded of his/her strength and capacity to survive. The permanent record forever reminds the survivor of the effects of child and adolescent sexual abuse, and facilitates the survivor's efforts to impact and educate others about this kind of trauma. The scars initially serve to promote the survivor's own physical, emotional, psychological, sexual, and social healing, but in the more advanced stages of healing, those scars also prompt the survivor to assist other abuse survivors in the community. They encourage the survivor to effect both personal and global change and healing. That means that even though you may want the abuse to be dealt with and put away, the survivor may need to keep it visible and accessible for some time.

While the process of healing spans the life cycle, the intensity does not remain constant. The survivor's process will probably follow a wave-like motion, in which he or she begins to experience greater and greater need for support and healing until an intense emotional peak is reached, when the intensity lessens and memories recede somewhat, and abuse issues are shelved for a time (until the need re-arises, and the emotions flare and so on and so forth...).

Survivors are most likely to invest their energy in managing abuse issues as they pass through major transitions in their lives. For instance, many survivors pop their first memories or opt for counseling when they begin life away from home (e.g. at college). Issues also commonly resurface upon the marriage or death of the perpetrator, when the perpetrator bears his/her own children, when the survivor marries or gives birth, and when the survivor's children or grandchildren reach the age when the survivor him- or herself was abused.

To put it more simply, while healing from sexual abuse takes a lifetime, sexual abuse need not always be on the forefront of your relationship with the survivor. Being a lover and a partner of a sexual abuse survivor is not for the faint of heart, but it can also be one of the most fulfilling and challenging relationships you may have. If you are unable to support the survivor in his/her healing process, take responsibility for your own limitations and help the survivor move on. If you're willing to try, good luck. Remember, those feelings of hopelessness and despair that you may have on rough days are temporary, but make sure you have the support you need for being a partner!

Psychological Impacts

Sometimes, those rough days become more and more frequent as the survivor struggles to heal and you strive to assist the survivor, as well as manage your own emotions. While therapy and support may enable you to avoid major psychological crises, it is possible that you may experience psychological impacts or symptoms in response to the survivor's disclosure and/or healing. Psychological effects include but are not limited to:

- denial of abuse
- repression or forgetting details of abuse following the disclosure
- minimization of abuse in order to avoid feelings generated by the disclosure
- projection of anger at the survivor (though the rage is experienced toward the perpetrator)
- emotional isolation and withdrawal
- depression (if you do not receive assistance or support, early signs of depression may become more serious and protracted (e.g. Major Depressive Episode, Dysthymia)
- constant focus or obsession with abuse
- repeated reexperiencing of the disclosure or inundation by images of the abuse (if you do not seek support early on, secondary Post-traumatic Stress Disorder may develop)

Just as it is important for the survivor to cope with his/her painful feelings and memories, it is important that you process your own experience. While some individuals choose to work through these feelings on their own, others opt for professional assistance. If your partner can provide you with support, and you have friends or relatives with whom you can share your feelings, then you may be able to manage without professional assistance. If your symptoms increase in their intensity, or if you find that you are unable to deal with the abuse and relationship issues, seek help from a therapist, trained in the area of sexual abuse. Not only is it important for you to maintain good mental health for yourself, but your continued self-esteem and emotional health enable you to act as an important ally for the survivor.

Exercise #42: "Recognizing psychological impacts"

Get a pen and some paper (or your journal). For the next 30 minutes, write about how things have been for you since you found out about the abuse. Don't concern yourself with punctuation, grammar, or logic, just write whatever comes to mind. Allow yourself to explore all of the feelings and reactions you've been having and express these on paper. Don't worry about knowing what to write, just do it!

When the 30 minutes are up, put your writing away and go do something else. Later, come back and read about the experiences you've been having. Allow yourself to learn about what you need, too.

Behavioral and Social Effects on the Partner

Just as you may experience physical, emotional, and psychological impacts following disclosure of abuse, your response may also include changes in behavior and social interaction. Changes may include but are not limited to:

- increased tearfulness or crying
- isolation and withdrawal
- increased need for alone time
- more frequent and intense expression of anger and rage, both at those who are present (e.g. non-protective parents) and those who are not (e.g. abuser)
- increase in attention-seeking behavior
- protectiveness and possessiveness toward survivor
- increased need to socialize with both survivor-partner couples, and non survivors (need for normalization and identification)
- researching effects of sexual abuse

Survivors and their partners endure many ups and downs and experience a myriad of changes in their lives independently and together. They may undergo these emotional and behavioral changes one at a time, or may experience general shifts in the way they relate to self and others. Doug describes his experience, which reflects one of the more common profiles maintained by lovers and survivors:

> *I met Drew just prior to his first big break, when he really dove headlong into his abuse issues. When he first started facing his memories, he had nightmares nearly every night, and flashbacks any time I tried to touch him. I reacted instinctually, trying to care for him, and soothe him, without touching him sexually. I listened to him night after night, and I handed him handkerchiefs when he needed them. It felt good to be close, even though we couldn't be together sexually.*

> *After the crisis passed, Drew stared to withdraw from me, and I got so confused. Here I'd been a part of everything, and then he started to shut me out. I felt so rejected, after having given him my all. I resented how he had taken from me, and then was ready to take off, without giving to me in return. I got resentful, and started going out more without him, and as soon as I did that, he got angry and threw me out. Then we were both alone and confused all over again.*

Doug aptly describes a pattern of mistrust and withdrawal that is common among lovers and survivors. In Doug and Drew's case, Doug was able to connect with Drew on a very intimate level during a period of intense emotional conflict and vulnerability. As soon as Drew regained some of his strength (and regained control of the emotional wall he maintained with others), he became scared and mistrustful of Doug's intimate "intrusion" into his life, no matter how helpful Doug had been. Because Drew did not discuss his feelings with Doug, Doug experienced Drew's withdrawal as an unfounded rejection, became distrustful of Drew and rejected him in turn. When Drew experienced Doug's rejection, he terminated the relationship completely, feeling that once again he'd been victimized.

Many survivors have an immensely difficult time trusting their partners and others in their support system. When others enter the personal realm of the survivor, the survivor does not differentiate between the violation of abuse, and the intimacy of a supportive relationship. The survivor distrusts his/her ally, which is experienced by the support provider or partner as an insult or rejection. The partner then reacts with rejection, and the cycle repeats itself until intervention is sought or until the survivor or partner terminates the relationship. This rejection further validates the survivor's negative self-image and beliefs that he/she is bad and deserves only abuse.

While this "testing" and distrusting is fairly common among survivors, this doesn't negate how frustrating, confusing, and maddening the experience may be. Try to talk things out with your partner in an honest, sensitive way, so that communication is restored during these chaotic times. Remember, too, that you have a right to your own health and happiness. You may need to ask yourself how much you are willing to do to keep the relationship going.

To assist your partner and maintain your own well-being, it will not only be important to understand the process which the two of you are going through, but also to get some assistance when the dynamics between the two of you become dysfunctional. It will become apparent that you need external support when any of the following is occurring:

- neither of you is communicating clearly and assertively with the other
- either one or both of you experience a sharp drop in self-esteem
- either one or both of you feel that your needs are not being met
- either of you is distrusting the other for no apparent reason
- either of you is responding aggressively or with hostility
- either of you is physically, emotionally, or sexually abusive

In addition to the impacts that disclosure of sexual abuse survival may have on the relationship, relationships outside the partnership may also be affected. Often, when a partner learns of incest within a family, he/she will encourage the survivor to confront his/her family. If the survivor is not ready or is unwilling to confront his/her family, the partner may choose to do it him- or herself. Unfortunately, this kind of reaction actually rescinds control from the survivor and generally leaves the survivor feeling helpless and victimized once again. It is important that you wait for the cues from the survivor, and respect the survivor's wishes even if it means that you contain or constrain your behavior until the survivor agrees to confront.

Exercise #43: "Recognizing behavioral and social impacts"

If your partner has already disclosed a history of abuse to you, has your behavior with your partner and others changed since the disclosure? What have you noticed about your needs to be separate from or connected with others? How has the expression of your feelings changed since the disclosure? Take some time and list the changes you've recognized in your behavior.

For the survivor and partner to share control in the relationship, the couple must follow the basic guidelines presented in the previous chapters. Most importantly, the relationship should be mutually consenting, there should be equality between the partners, each should respect the needs and desires of the other, trust should be developed prior to sexually intimate contact, and each partner should feel safe and secure within the relationship. Beyond these guidelines, the partners must trust their instincts and develop creative ways to support and challenge each other. This will likely include meeting the following needs:

Needs of the Lover/Survivor Couple
- Each must make an effort to understand and validate the experience of the other. This may include reading or talking to others about these experiences.
- Each must make an effort to communicate honestly and assertively with the other.
- Each should encourage the other to express emotions in an open and healthy fashion.

- Each should be free to ask the other questions, and each should have the right to refuse to answer questions as he/she feels necessary
- The couple must explore open avenues of sexuality and develop a repertoire of sexual behaviors that are experienced by both as healthy, safe, and non-exploitative. Positive sexuality should be reinforced for both partners.
- The couple must share control within the relationship. This will be promoted by active participation in healing by both survivor and partner.

While most support providers would agree that all couples must come up with their own way to manage their relationship, the basic guidelines listed in this book may at least provide a foundation for the couple. Christine Courtois, author of *Healing the Incest Wound*, has written a comprehensive set of "instructions" for managing a disclosure of past child sexual abuse. While each partner must decide for him- or herself what he/she is capable of offering to his/her partner, this list offers some helpful, straightforward responses which can be used when a disclosure is made. Dr. Courtois' ideas are provided below in their full original form:

How to Respond to a Disclosure of Past Child Sexual Abuse

- "Be open to the disclosure. Let the survivor know you are open to discussing what she feels comfortable telling you about her past.
- Appreciate how difficult it is to make a disclosure and to confide long-held secrets.
- Offer her support and understanding. Empathize with her without pitying her. Let her know that you hurt to hear that she had such difficult events to contend with.

- Strive to be sensitive but matter-of-fact in your initial response rather than highly emotional. Know that she needs a calm, accepting, encouraging response.
- Encourage her to tell you details as she chooses and as she is able. Don't press for details and don't focus on the sexual details. It may suffice for her to tell you only the most minimal of details or she might want you to know more. It is her decision, to do as she is able.
- Don't blame her. Emphasize that, no matter what the circumstance, she was not to blame. Be careful of questions that sound blaming, such as "Didn't you try to stop it?" "Did you tell him that you didn't like it?" "How did you know your mother wouldn't believe you if you didn't try to tell her?" "Maybe you really did enjoy it."
- Don't try to deny that it happened and don't tell her to forget it and go on with her life or otherwise "talk the abuse into going away." It's not "all in her head" and she needs to know that she is believed and supported. Don't tell her she made it up to get attention or "things like that just don't happen in good families," etc. It is especially tempting to deny incest when the perpetrator is a respected and loved member of the family and/or a "pillar of the community."
- Allow her to have her emotions and expect that she will have positive as well as negative feelings or that her predominant ones might be confusion and ambivalence. Not uncommonly, survivors have a feeling of warmth and love toward the perpetrator for the non-exploitative parts of their relationship especially if he was the only family member to offer her nurturance.
- Don't respond with panic. Allow yourself some time to sort out your feelings.

- Don't pressure her and don't try to rush her. She needs to make choices and take action at her discretion. She will also heal at her own pace. Unfortunately, the recovery process is often lengthy—she needs support over its duration.
- Encourage her to seek therapy if she has not yet done so. Let her know that there are professionals who specialize in treating the aftereffects of abuse and who can help her. Offer her hope that she can recover from the effects of the past.
- Encourage her to make choices that are in her best interest. Don't try to stop her from making choices and don't make them for her.
- Don't attempt to be overprotective or rescue her and don't confront the perpetrator or other family members without her knowledge and permission. Be aware that angry and retaliatory behavior can hurt her by making her feel anxious, out of control, and powerless.
- Talk to her about taking action to safeguard children in the family if the perpetrator still poses a risk. Other disclosures and reporting might be necessary. Indicate your support and willingness to explore possible avenues of action.
- Don't treat her like "damaged or spoiled goods" following disclosure. If you are her sexual partner, she needs assurance that she is still lovable and attractive. Try to maintain your normal level of sexual interaction and don't try to "make everything better with sex." Seek out professional assistance or a support group if your feelings are strongly negative or you find yourself obsessing about the details of abuse rather than focusing on the welfare of your partner. It is appropriate to share your feelings of anger, hurt, etc., but be sure they are

directed toward the perpetrator and the
abuse and are not blaming of the survivor.

- Follow up with her after her initial disclosure
to you. Don't let the disclosure 'go down a
black hole,' never to be mentioned again.
And, don't tell her that you forgot that she
had ever made a disclosure to you.
- Maintain your normal expression of affection
with the survivor. Touching, holding and
hugging can be especially comforting. If you
do not have a relationship with the survivor
which normally includes physical contact,
ask her permission before making any and
respect her wishes.
- Support her in future disclosures, confrontations or reporting. Be aware that this may
be especially difficult for other family
members, who are bound to feel split
loyalty and to get caught up in other family
roles and interaction patterns.
- Respect her privacy. Do not break her confidence and don't discuss her disclosure
without her permission."[11]

Although I have attempted to provide basic information on
the impacts of sexual abuse on the survivor, the partner, and
the relationship, there are always questions which remain
unanswered. After reviewing this material, I asked survivors and
their partners what questions they wanted to have answered.
Their responses appear in the next chapter. Hopefully, you may
find responses to some of your own unanswered questions in
the pages that follow.

Section III

Asking For Help And Using It
To Your Benefit

After reading the last seven chapters, your head may be spinning. You have a lot of information now, but you may still feel a little confused. You may have questions that are still unanswered and feel uncertain about how to put this all together for a relationship that works. And, even if you feel like you have a handle on the information, you may still have concerns that need to be addressed more personally.

The next few chapters answer common questions asked by partners, they offer some basic ideas for managing your relationship, and they provide resources for both you and your partner. If you finish this book and want more information, select one of the books in Chapter 10, or locate a conference or a group for partners. You have been courageous to get this far, don't stop now.

Chapter 8
Your Questions Answered

Physical

"Whose body is this anyway?"

Many people wonder about the effects which sexual abuse has on the physical being: the body. Those effects may be obvious at the time of the abuse, and may also be reflected years later. Here are some of the common questions about the effects of sexual abuse on the survivor and his/her body:

Will my partner ever become comfortable with her body? What I can do to make it easier for her?

The degree to which the survivor becomes comfortable with her body really depends on who she is and what she's been through. Some survivors come away from the abuse feeling OK about their bodies, even though they are emotionally devastated. Research suggests that when victims are able to resist, struggle, or say "No!" they are less likely to feel betrayed by their bodies, and have less trouble with physical memories and symptoms. The majority of survivors experience some difficulty with body image and comfort.

The degree to which a survivor experiences discomfort may also reflect the level of healing she is in. Most survivors go through phases of healing: from identifying the abuse issues, to talking about what happened, to experiencing old emotions, to confronting abusers and non-protective parents, to integrating memories, and finally to healing sexuality. While the survivor may become less comfortable with her body during some of the earlier phases, it is likely that she will gain comfort with her body in later phases, especially when the focus is on healing her sexuality.

Although your partner is the only one who can determine how comfortable she is with her body, you can help her feel more positive about herself. Respect her feelings, but don't be afraid to reality test with her. When your partner says, "My body will always be ugly and dirty," you can be supportive, but objective. If your partner's body is of average size and shape, you can point out that you understand that she feels ugly and dirty, but that, in fact, her body does not look any different than the average woman's body. If you think that her body is beautiful, tell her so! Remember, it is important to validate her feelings, even if reality suggests a different perception. If you consider your partner's body ugly, it probably won't be helpful to admit this, but your partner might feel comforted if you identify one of her better qualities. For instance, if you can identify some of the qualities which attracted you to your partner in the first place, you might say, "I know you're unhappy with the way you look right now, but you have other great qualities. I fell in love with your sense of humor and your sensitivity."

When your partner begins to work on healing her sexuality, she will probably need some time on her own to discover her body. When she becomes more comfortable with her own body, she may invite you to explore with her. As much as you may want to guide her and show her how much you care for her, it will be important to go at her pace, and to follow her lead. As the sexual trust grows between the two of you, you will learn to share yourselves, and the control of your intimacy.

Why does my girlfriend try to hide her femininity by wearing androgynous or "neutral" clothing?

Many survivors fear their sexuality. Survivors often believe that it is their sexuality which has caused the abuse to happen: that in some way, being female elicited the abuse by the perpetrator. Many abuse survivors detach themselves from those qualities and characteristics which they associate with their gender. Male survivors may take care to hide their attractive physical attributes: if the survivor has been complemented on the size of his penis or the shape of his buttocks, he may choose to wear baggy pants that hide those body parts. If the female survivor feels that she has been assaulted because of her femininity, she may cut her hair short, wear loose-fitting clothes to hide her breasts, or even change the shape of her body by dieting or overeating.

If the survivor believes that he/she has been victimized because of his/her young age, the survivor may try to appear older, by wearing makeup or more adult clothing. Conversely, if the survivor believes that he/she has been abused because he/she looked "old enough," then the survivor may attempt to look younger. Survivors may wear hairstyles that make them appear more youthful, wear clothing that is more juvenile, even act like younger children, including playing childhood games, sucking their thumbs, or wetting the bed. There is a fairly large percentage of female survivors who become anorexic, starving themselves so that they loose their secondary sex characteristics: these survivors believe that, without breasts, or other sensual curves, they appear to be little girls, and are no longer vulnerable to the adult male (unfortunately, the sex offender may not be deterred by the changed physical form).

In addition to the survivor's fear of and discomfort with his/her own sexuality, survivors are often apprehensive about "being in the spotlight." Abuse survivors may believe that something about them "stood out," attracted the abuser to them for some unknown reason. Survivors were noticed, and then they were violated. The logic of the survivor may be as simple as that: if you stand out, others will see you, and if you are noticed, you will be hurt/punished. The incest survivor learns to fade into the background in his/her own family, he/she learns how to hide in his/her own home: his/her survival begins to depend on invisibility.

The abuse survivor may use clothing to help him/her fit in and fade out, wearing neutral clothing that hides all of his/her curves, but also blends in with those around him/her. He/she may wear hairstyles that hides his/her face, or complies with the current trend (so as not to look different from the rest). In school, the survivor may learn to be "part of the gang," and may opt to steer clear of positions of leadership or status. He/she may be an unremarkable student so that even the teacher will not notice him/her. At work, the survivor's "invisible trend" may continue: he/she may be a steady employee, but may rarely excel at his/her job. Socially, he/she may know his/her colleagues, but may not actually develop relationships with anyone. Even in marriage, the survivor may take a backseat to his/her partner, fading in to the woodwork, so that he/she can continue to be invisible and safe. A prime example of the invisible survivor is the consummate "Doctor's wife": the woman who everyone sees at the social functions on the arm of her husband, but whom no one really knows, because she is unimportant; she is simply an extension of her prominent husband. She is safe behind her role and social facade, vulnerable to no one, because she is invisible.

I can't seem to tease my wife about her body without her flipping out! Why is she so hyper-sensitive?

For most survivors, having the body noticed is associated with abuse. In many cases of sexual abuse, the perpetrator may have begun to abuse the child or adolescent by noticing and remarking about her body. The perpetrator may also have teased the child during the abuse, taunting her about the size of her breasts or buttocks, pinching or tickling her skin or genitals, or even physically torturing the child's body to gain compliance. During adulthood, even playful teasing may elicit fearful or hostile responses from the survivor. Survivors cope with their abuse by learning to be hypervigilant, or supersensitive, to everything around them, in order to predict abusive and non-abusive situations. As the survivor becomes hyper-sensitive about her own body, she may react to remarks about her body as if the comments were physical threats or violations.

In addition to the survivor's memories and associations with being teased in the past, she may carry a lot of shame about her body, and may perceive herself as ugly or "damaged." As a result, it may be difficult for the survivor to believe that her partner can accept this "damaged" part of her, and that she will not be rejected for her physical "flaws." The survivor may have come to believe that she will be rejected as soon as her partner notices the "damage," whether it takes him/her days, months, or years. Even playful teasing may be interpreted by the survivor as a form of rejection by her partner.

Is it common for survivors to develop physical symptoms of personal injury when they are exploring incidents of child sexual abuse? It seems my partner has developed many somatic problems since the first memory "popped."

There are a number of reasons for the development of physical problems or symptoms following the recognition that abuse has occurred. First, the very act of remembering may require a tremendous amount of the survivor's energy. While we are beginning to understand how memory works, we do not yet know how abuse memories are "forgotten" and later restored.

It may be helpful to use the following analogy: a child victim may be unable to manage his/her memories of the abuse at the time that he/she is being abused. The child creates a safe or lock box inside his/her brain that only he/she can open. When the survivor feels uncomfortable or insecure with the memory of the abuse, he/she opens the safe and places the memory inside. He/she carefully locks it away and prohibits the memory from entering his/her consciousness. The survivor may continue to do this with painful feelings, images or memories until the lock box is full, or until the survivor decides that he/she no longer wants to hide these feelings and thoughts from him/herself. Sometimes, the survivor is unaware of deciding to stop the process, but may have developed an intimate relationship in which he/she feels safe enough to stop (and the decision is made unconsciously). At that point, new memories are no longer stuffed, and old memories and images begin to re-emerge into consciousness (sometimes after many decades).

The act of unlocking the safe requires tremendous energy from the survivor. And, while managing all of the new and old memories also requires a great deal of energy from the survivor, the release of information also frees up all of the energy used to keep the safe locked. This exchange of energies may leave the survivor feeling emotionally and physically exhausted! When the survivor must continue to manage his/her current lifestyle, while coping with old emotions and images, it is likely that he/she will develop symptoms of depression and physical illness. Both force the survivor to slow down and nourish him/herself, and enable the survivor to take the process more slowly.

A secondary result of this process is that as the survivor opens up the hidden part of him/herself, he/she may become more open to his/her body on the whole. Prior to the releasing of memories, the survivor may have kept his/her body "dead" or numb to physical pain or pleasure. As the safe is unlocked, the survivor is likely to become more aware of his/her bodily sensations. While the survivor may have been a real trooper in the past when it came to physical pain or illness, he/she may actually recognize pain and discomfort to a greater degree once the lock box has been opened (some survivors even go through a phase of hypochondria when they first gain body awareness. After years of feeling numb, the experience of physical discomfort or even minor pain can be confusing and frightening). Most survivors require some time and experience to get used to their new, sensitive boundaries.

In addition to the physical symptoms associated with releasing or "popping" memories, there are physical symptoms associated with the emotions, images, and memories which resurface. When a survivor does not retrieve visual memories, he/she may experience "body memories," which remind the survivor of the abuse using physical signals from the past. For instance, a survivor whose testicles were fondled repeatedly might experience a tingling or "brushing" sensation in his genitals at times when his attention is otherwise diverted from his sexuality. A female survivor might feel someone reach from behind her to squeeze her breasts or buttocks, even though no one is with her. Survivors frequently have body memories of being penetrated, especially at the times of day when the abuse originally occurred (many survivors have reported body memories during a semi-sleep state.

Survivors "come to" after a deep sleep, experiencing pressure on their chests, and the pain of penetration in the genitals or anus. It is probable that these memories emerge during the sleep cycle, because original abuse was also endured during early morning hours. These memories may be considered state-dependent).

Even when the survivor is able to retrieve visual memories, he/she may reexperience the physical pain of the original abuse. Some survivors have "flashbacks" and actually reexperience the abusive situation. If the survivor is flashing on a gang rape while he/she is sleeping with his/her partner, he/she may fear the partner, as well as other "hallucinated" figures. The survivor may thrash about, as if being victimized, and may feel pain in all of his/her body parts. The pain, though archaic, is real, and may even leave physical damage in its wake: while the survivor described above will probably not require medical attention, if the flashback is severe enough, the survivor may injure him/herself during the flashback, as a result of lashing out at perceived rapists, or even from trying to escape from his/her own genitalia.

Why does my boyfriend sweat profusely, grind his teeth and toss constantly when he sleeps?

Fitful sleep is often a sign of active dreaming. The dream state is considered by many therapists to be a time when the individual can think about ideas and situations that he/she refuses to think about during the wake state. Some people generate fantasies while they sleep and allow themselves to try things that they might not otherwise try. Other people dream about harming those who hurt them. And still others use sleep in order to solve the problems which have arisen during the work day and have not been resolved.

Survivors dream as non-survivors dream. One major difference between the dream state of the survivor and that of the non-survivor is that the survivor may be trying to resolve a problem that has no resolution: survivors frequently struggle with images of the original abuse, unable to loose these pictures from their minds. During sleep, survivors may reenter the abuse situation, determined to change the course of history, but generally survivors reenter the image alone, and as children, vulnerable once again to the abuse. They may toss and turn as they try to avoid the mouth or genitals of the abuser in the dream, may gnash their teeth as they try to keep out unwanted objects, or may cry out as they try to protect themselves. The amount of energy in accomplishing these acts can cause an increase in heart rate and blood pressure, labored breathing, flushed color, and perspiration.

Cognitive
"Will we ever stop thinking about this?"

Most partners ask this question sooner or later. Dealing with sexual abuse takes a lot out of the survivor, the partner, and the relationship. It also provides challenge, and an opportunity to ask questions that might never be raised. Still, that doesn't mean that you want to spend your entire life asking and answering those same questions! Sexual abuse never goes away, but the intensity of the issues fade as they are dealt with and integrated. Issues resurface at times of stress and transition, generally with great intensity which wanes fairly quickly after the issues are addressed. As was noted in the last section, sexual abuse leaves its physical traces, but it also impacts how the survivor thinks. Some of the common questions about the thought processes of the survivor follow:

*Will my partner always be stuck in the past?
Will she ever learn to look forward to the times
ahead?*

As uncomfortable as it is for both survivor and partner, looking backwards and confronting the issues of the past are part of the healing process. If the survivor is actively engaged in the healing process and the partner is offering support for this work, there is no reason for the survivor to remain forever "stuck."

There probably isn't anything inherently helpful or good about focusing on the past, yet, when the survivor is able to deal with the past, by reviewing and confronting it, she can emotionally defuse the memories, and put the energy bound up with past issues to better use. The energy freed by reopening up historic abuse issues can be used to create new ideas, behaviors, and feelings. The survivor's temporary emphasis on the past enables her to create a future for herself and her partner. Confrontation, healing and growth all take time, so patience is a must for both survivor and partner.

*Sometimes my boyfriend obsesses for long
periods of time about the abuse. What's done is
done, so why does he go on about this stuff?*

The scars left behind by sexual abuse last forever. Even though therapy may enable the survivor to move forward in his life, nothing can take away the fact that he survived a tremendous trauma. To keep going, the survivor learned different techniques and coping skills, some of which were more helpful, effective and healthy than others.

One cognitive, or mental, coping strategy commonly used by survivors is a form of focusing. Often, during the abuse, children learn to focus on some other thought or image to avoid experiencing the pain. As the survivor becomes more and more skilled with this strategy, he may learn that he can tune everything out quite easily.

The problem is that the survivor may begin to use this strategy whenever he feels uncomfortable or experiences any emotions at all. As soon as the survivor begins to feel physical changes that he associates with surfacing emotions (such as a lump in the throat, or tears welling up, or "butterflies" in the stomach), he starts to tune out and focus on some minute detail. He totally contains the emotion by avoiding experiencing it at all.

When the survivor uses this strategy as his primary or only coping device, he may become obsessive. As was noted in Chapter 3, obsessing on a thought is a way to avoid feeling anxious, upset or angry. It allows the individual to totally follow his head, and forget his heart altogether. When emotions become overwhelming or too frequent to manage, the survivor may develop Obsessive Compulsive Disorder. In this case, obsessions may fail to stop the feelings which arise, and the survivor may need to create compulsive behaviors to bind or contain those feelings. Unfortunately, most find that neither the obsessions nor the compulsions liberate them from their overwhelming emotions, and often these runaway thoughts and behaviors prohibit them from living a normal life.

When the survivor finally seeks help, he is usually trained to identify the thought that precedes the compulsive behavior. When the thoughts can be accurately identified, they are analyzed and broken down. The survivor learns to discard thoughts that are not realistic and replace them with logical, healthy thoughts. The survivor learns to analyze his thoughts to identify feelings that are managed by obsessive thinking. Then, the therapist and survivor work through these feelings together, the therapist training the survivor to finally experience the overwhelming feelings rather than mentally running from them. Most survivors find that once they are able to confront their fear of emoting (at all), they find themselves to be more capable and relaxed.

> *Everything seems so black or white to my partner. Is there a way for him to stop focusing on the extremes?*

Children who are abused often crave an explanation for what is happening to them. Because no healthy explanation is available, child survivors create their own rationale. As most survivors hate the experience of helplessness, they seek a way to assume some control over the abuse. Taking responsibility for the abuse, by reasoning that he/she somehow deserves the abuse, allows the child to feel more in control (at the sacrifice of self-esteem). Unfortunately, by assuming control in this way, the child begins to see himself as all bad. Children who are not abused, or are treated with respect and fairness are then viewed as all good.

While the survivors uses this strategy or style of thinking effectively while the abuse is occurring, it becomes obsolete once the abuse has been terminated. This extreme thinking is non-rational and distorted, and may leave the survivor feeling unhappy and helpless (contrary to its purpose!).

For the survivor to think more rationally, it is important that he learn to analyze his thoughts and determine how realistic they are. When an individual focuses on the extremes, its often helpful for him to do a reality check. When Sam turns to his wife and says, "This relationship is totally worthless," he might want to find some evidence for this assertion. For instance, Sam might want to review the conversations that he and his wife have had over the years to determine if there has ever been a conversation that was helpful or soothing. He might also want to review all of the components of their relationship in order to determine if each part is negative or if there are some positive qualities that he has failed to recognize (during the heat of the battle). Finally, it's important that Sam learn to deal with "percentages." For example, when making an "extreme" statement, Sam can step back and ask himself, "What percentage of this relationship is healthy and what percentage is unhealthy?" When Sam can find even one percent which is good, the situation can't be considered all bad.

Changing the way you think is hard work, and the partner must be willing to support the survivor in his efforts. If you, too, think in distorted or unrealistic ways, seek some assistance for yourself, or buddy up with your partner and work on healthy cognitive functioning together!

Why does my girlfriend think that everything I do or say his directed at her?

Survivors come in all different shapes and sizes, with a variety of personal characteristics. They share many common qualities, including an often rigid or controlled way of thinking and an intense self-focus.

There are many reasons why an individual may focus on herself. Survivors often learn to turn their focus inwards during the abuse, in order to withdraw from the intolerable, and also to assume what little control they can over the situation.

The experiences of both Beth and Melanie in Chapter 3 demonstrate the survivor's need to use the internal locus of control in order to manage the abusive situation.

While both of these women endured horrendous traumas, they were able to shift their focus inwards and temporarily mentally deny the threat posed by their abusers. Instead, they concentrated on controlling as many aspects of the abuse as they could. Beth found that she was able to control where she was raped, while Melanie controlled the site of the pain she experienced (she bit herself in order to focus on that pain rather than that generated by her abuser). This ability to focus on the self, rather than on extraneous details, served as a coping mechanism for each woman. As the abuse ends and the survivor works to move on with her life, she must find a way to rid herself of the obsolete coping strategies (that were once useful during the abuse) and to develop healthier skills.

In addition to the self-focus which the survivor develops in response to the abuse, there may be other, less direct sources of self-focus. When the survivor comes from an incestuous home, or when parents are perceived as non-protective or emotionally abusive, the survivor may fail to thrive as an individual. In order for the child to develop a complete sense of self, it is important that she feel good about herself, and have access to successful, nurturing role models.

When the child is instead faced with abusive parents, or those who are unable to function as caretakers or guardians, she must search for other adults to look up to. If she is unable to find someone to build her self-esteem and to offer her goals to which she can aspire, her sense of self will not develop fully. She will experience these voids in her sense of worth and being and may feel intimidated by others who are more self-assured. In order to hide the personal voids she experiences, she may become passive and "invisible" to others or she may become quite egocentric or self-focused. When the child feels intimidated or helpless around others, she is likely to focus on herself in order to maintain what little sense of control she does have. Should that control or self-focus be taken away, the child is likely to feel threatened, helpless and frightened. When the child whose sense of self is already tenuous, is abused, the need to control outweighs all else. This survivor may mature into a rigid, sometimes overbearing individual who has difficulty trusting others. She is likely to be overwhelmed easily and may continuously search for those who help her feel strong and successful. Should she be unable to find supportive others, she may become even more solitary and narcissistic.

> *My husband constantly loses his train of thought when talking with me about his abuse issues. Is this normal?*

Most survivors don't want to remember anything about their abuse. These memories are painful and require considerable energy to manage and explore. It is common for survivors to "forget" their abuse, sometimes even as it happened, in order to endure. The urge to deny may work comprehensively or it may work selectively. A survivor may retain some memories and forget others, or may completely wipe out all knowledge of the abuse.

When a survivor is disclosing, the shame and emotional distress can be overwhelming. In fact, the emotions generated during disclosure may match those of the original abuse, setting off that same mechanism of denial. Memories may be temporarily "lost" during disclosure as a result of the shame associated with the abuse, or due to denial elicited by overwhelming emotions.

Robert, a chronic incest survivor and sex addict, was famous in group therapy for losing his train of thought. During his first year in group, he spent a fair amount of time talking about his "conquests," rather than focusing on his abuse issues. He listened attentively when others were speaking, but it was hard to tell how much was actually sinking in. Finally, Robert began to tell his story. He'd start the session tearfully, talking about holiday dinners, a time when sexual abuse was guaranteed. And, as his focus on the meal intensified, his tears would dry and he would encourage the group to talk about favorite foods and whatnot. After several attempts, another member finally confronted Robert and asked if the food was all Robert recalled about those times. Robert looked around the group, confused, and said, "You mean I didn't tell you about what happened under the table?" The selective memory allowed this survivor, like many others to endure the abuse, and the disclosure. In Robert's case, the memories were so painful that his ability to disclose the information was limited to spotty recollection.

Behavioral
"Can we do to undo?"

Many partners have a difficult time managing the most obvious correlates of sexual abuse: the often unhealthy behavior that they see in the survivors with whom they interact. When a survivor is ingesting drugs or alcohol in order to forget his/her memories or is physically hurting him/herself, the partner may not be able to "look the other way." These behaviors cry out for intervention, they alert the partner that something must be done. What about the more subtle things that happen? What about the intense focus on the abuse issues, the controlling attitude, the need for cleanliness or the desire to be separate? How much should a partner insist on? What can a partner expect? Is there anything a partner can actually do to help the survivor heal? And, what can the survivor do? Does it ever go away? Some of these issues are addressed below:

> *Is there something I can do for my partner to help her get over these sexual abuse issues? Is there a way to help her behave more normally?*

Unfortunately, sexual abuse never goes away. At best, it is worked through and integrated, so that the survivor can forever honor her ability to survive and overcome. The emotional scars are permanent and may be difficult for both survivor and partner to accept.

When the survivor has yet to deal with the abuse issues, her attitude and behavior may be stormy. The untapped emotions are likely to eat away at her and cause her to behave in ways that she might not otherwise behave. During this period, the survivor needs much emotional support to manage the past, present and future. And, because it is important that the survivor have an ally and a guide in her exploration of past trauma (so that she is not helpless and alone once again), the partner can support the survivor by encouraging her to seek professional assistance. While the partner may want to be everything to the survivor and support her completely, it is impossible for the partner to act as the survivor's therapist as well. Generally this leads to decline in the health of both partners and in the relationship.

When the survivor has entered therapy and is dealing with her issues, she needs support for her therapeutic efforts, but also needs support for living a healthy life. When the survivor is having a particularly difficult time in therapy, it is important that the partner nurture and support her, encouraging the survivor to cope in ways that are healthy. For instance, instead of enabling the survivor to withdraw and isolate, the partner can encourage the survivor to share and disclose. When the survivor is immersed in the helplessness of the past, the partner can assist the survivor by helping her to take a break to feel powerful in the present, for example by working out with the survivor or by helping her to feel productive. Finally, when the survivor needs to relax and be soothed, and has relied on alcohol or sexual addiction in the past (for example), the partner can offer to draw a bubble bath for the survivor or invite her on a peaceful walk. Partners can set healthy examples, and provide support for the survivor who wishes to lead a more functional, normal and relaxed lifestyle.

> *I think that my partner has been abused but he says he doesn't remember anything happening. What are some of the typical signs and symptoms that continue to show up even during adulthood?*

Even when a survivor has no visual memories of being abused in the past, he may sense that something has happened. In addition, he may do or say things that make others suspect a history of sexual abuse.

Many of the effects of sexual abuse are outlined in Chapter 2, but are also summarized briefly here. While each individual who has been sexually abused responds somewhat differently, most survivors generally develop a coping style that emphasizes control over self and others, or one which reflects complete passivity. Survivors then, may become "doormats" for others to use and walk on, or conversely, may demand respect and power during their interactions.

Survivors who were forced to submit during early violation and abuse may continue to be submissive when confronted by those with authority and power. Male survivors who remain submissive from the time of the abuse may choose sexual identities in which they are forced to be receptive or submissive. The survivor may choose a homosexual lifestyle if he was abused by a man, in order to continue submitting. If shows of strength or self-esteem were punished by the perpetrator, the survivor may resist acting this way again, even when there is a good chance that he will be rewarded for such behavior.

If the male survivor chooses to lead a heterosexual lifestyle, he may act passively in his intimate relationships, never making the first move, especially during sexual interaction. If the survivor has made peace with his sexual identity, but still chooses a passive behavioral style, he may select a career in which he is employed by someone else, and receives little appreciation for his efforts. He may complain about his work situation, but will resist leaving the familiar, exploitative environment. If the survivor functions well at work and at home, his personal style may reflect passivity or "weakness." He may perceive himself as effeminate or "nerdish," may believe himself to be incapable of household repairs or chores, and may choose activities which require more brain than brawn. These qualities in themselves need not indicate that the individual is a survivor, but coupled with other behaviors, thoughts, feelings (e.g. of low self-esteem, shame, rage), and memories can provide a more accurate identification of the male survivor.

Another role which survivors may portray is the controlled, power-hungry individual. When a person has been victimized and violated, he is left feeling helpless and confused. If that individual has developed a sense of wholeness, completeness, or self-worth prior to the abuse, then it is likely that he will fight these feelings for the rest of his life, probably by developing a very empowered, controlling identity.

These survivors grow up hypervigilant, or supersensitive to everything around them. They gather more information than others in their environment, often developing their intellect in the process. They maintain their composure at all costs, and rarely let others in on their inner workings. They detest feeling vulnerable or helpless (e.g. and often associate these feelings with "weakness"), and may, restrict their range of emotions. They enjoy being in positions of authority and often choose positions such as Manager or CEO. While they may be uncomfortable in the limelight, they take pleasure in running things from behind closed doors (e.g. like the Wizard of Oz).

Those survivors who actively maintain control of self and others may choose homosexual or heterosexual identities (some portion of this depends on whether they believed themselves to be homosexual prior to the abuse). Those that choose homosexual identities are likely to take a more dominant role in their relationships and may even opt for sado-masochistic relationships. Those that select heterosexual lifestyles may emphasize control over their partners, behave possessively, and may appear to be very traditional and even sexist. Whether the survivor leads a homosexual or heterosexual lifestyle, he may be hyper sexual (i.e. he may respond to most situations with sexual behavior) and may even develop a sexual addiction. He may spend extensive periods of time attracting partners, flirting with partners, sexually acting out, or fantasizing about sexual interactions (through imagination, erotica, pornography or fetishes).

While male survivors do react to sexual abuse somewhat differently than female survivors, there are some characteristics and qualities that are common among all survivors. Memories of childhood are generally vague or splotchy, especially during the period in which the child or adolescent was abused. Emotions such as sadness, rage and shame are always close to the surface in the survivor, and may flare up at any time, in response to even the slightest problem. Survivors rarely want to discuss or explore their emotions, especially if the abuse issues have not yet been recognized. Survivors tend to be independent, even "loners," and may require very little interaction with others (or they may be personally demanding and may want your attention all the time). Sexuality is either extremely prominent, even to the point of promiscuity, or may fade into the background.

If you suspect that your partner has been abused, but has not disclosed to you about his past, be nurturing and caring and ask him directly. If he does not remember a history of abuse, you might suggest that he seek counseling to explore his past a bit, or do some reading of survivor literature to determine if he identifies with any of the concepts discussed. If he is unwilling to make an effort to explore or identify his issues, respect his decision. Should he engage in self-destructive or dangerous behaviors, confront him with your concerns and suggest again that he seek professional assistance.

Sometimes I come home and find my girlfriend hurting herself. It scares me. What can I do?

Self-mutilation and self-destructive behavior are common behavioral responses to the painful emotions often experienced by sexual abuse survivors. And, as much as all support providers need to respond to the seriousness of these actions (depending on the lethality of her behavior, you may even need to hospitalize her), you can't watch the survivor all the time. She is the one who ultimately must decide to stop harming herself.

There is a multitude of reasons why survivors choose to hurt themselves. Bridget offers some insight into her self-mutilation:

> *I started to cut myself when I just couldn't stand being numb anymore. I was used to walking through crowds, without ever sensing that others were around me. I was used to not feeling my clothes on my body. It was OK that I couldn't feel my feet hit the carpet or the sidewalk. When I met Anne, I wanted so badly to be able to heal my body. I want to feel the softness of her hand rubbing my back. I want to experience how gentle her touch was on my face and my body, and wanted to feel the connection with her. And, damn it if I couldn't! There just wasn't anything. I couldn't feel even the touches I longed for. One day, in my frustration, I wanted to see if I could make my body feel anything, even if extreme, even if painful. When that razor sliced into my skin, and I saw the blood run down my arm, I actually felt it. It hurt, but I felt something. Something was better than nothing at all.*

This numbness may be limited to physical feelings, or it may encompass the survivor's sense of her life. The survivor may feel that she is floating through her life, failing to actually make an impact, unable to feel alive. When this is the case, the survivor may begin to cut herself in order to determine whether she really is alive, validated by the sign of blood coursing through her veins, even if the process causes her physical pain.

Other survivors cut, burn, disfigure and amputate in order to punish themselves. These survivors manage the shame they experience about the sexual abuse, but repenting, trying to remove the "dirty" or "damaged" part in order to once again be clean and pure. Unfortunately, survivors who maim themselves find repeatedly that nothing, not even their penance, can remove the emotional scars of sexual abuse. These survivors are able to actually accomplish their actions (most of us would probably pass out if we tried to burn our arms with cigarettes, pull out our pubic hairs, or cut out our genitalia, for example) by dissociating or mentally separating mind from body. They begin to perceive their bodies and body parts as separate entities, to be used or abused without harm to the rest of the self. Unfortunately, the dissociative process enables the survivor to harm herself, but does not prevent her from requiring serious medical care. Even if she didn't physically feel the pain involved with cutting her inner thigh open, the survivor may still bleed to death.

Self-mutilation is a very serious sign of sexual abuse survival. If the survivor is not yet receiving counseling, get her assistance now. If she will not go, bring assistance to her, via ambulance or home health care. While it is important not to reward the survivor for her self-mutilation (by providing her with attention and support only when she hurts herself), it is important to take this behavior seriously and respond to it as the life-threatening action that it may be. While most survivors who self-mutilate may not actually intend to kill themselves, accidents do happen.

> *My partner spends a lot of time trying to please me. I'm all for the royal, nurture treatment, but she never spends any energy on her own needs and interests. Do other survivors act this way?*

Survivors aren't the only folks who put the needs of others before their own. In particular, those individuals who are raised

184 • S. Yvette de Beixedon, Ph.D.

in very traditional, patriarchal homes, are often taught to serve their husbands and brothers first and foremost. Those who are raised with conservative religious beliefs, often learn that to serve others is the way of God, even if it requires great sacrifice on the part of the "giver." In families in which there is an alcoholic parent, children assume adult responsibilities in order to "cover" for the alcoholic, often taking on tasks beyond their level of capability.

Similarly, in the incestuous home, the abused child learns that she is invisible and worthless unless she is serving the needs of the perpetrator. To act in any other way is to elicit punishment, generally in the form of further sexual abuse. This being the case, the survivor generally learns to remain compliant and to serve the perpetrator at all costs. Even when the survivor escapes the incestuous family, her compliance and martyrdom continue, as her original fear of punishment and rejection are maintained. Her needs are rarely identified or met, as she employs all of her energies into meeting the needs of her partner. If the partner is very self-focused and manipulative (a "user" or "taker"), the co-dependent behavior will be maintained. If the survivor is lucky or becoming healthier in her selection of partners, the partner will resist the survivor's co-dependent subservience and as that the survivor begin to identify and meet her own needs.

My partner started counseling for her abuse issues a short while ago. As they have begun to work more deeply, my partner has become more and more anxious about therapy. Recently, she started taking anti-anxiety pills before her sessions to overcome some of her terror. Is this OK, or is it important that she experience her fears without medication?

The needs and capabilities of each survivor are different. Some can withstand intense pain and anxiety, while others emotionally and physically shut down after brief bouts of distress and anger. Therapy for sexual abuse survival is a difficult process which requires a lot of energy from both survivor and therapist.

The survivor must be willing to learn to become vulnerable

with the therapist, to explore her memories, thoughts, and feelings. She must commit to interacting with her therapist in session, and to confronting the feelings which are elicited by the interaction itself. For instance, sometimes the physical features or mannerisms of the therapist remind the survivor of someone from the past, maybe even the perpetrator. In some cases, the survivor seeks an alternative therapist, but for the most part, the survivor and therapist work together to explore the thoughts and fears which arise in response to the therapist. Often, as they work together, the frightening resemblances disappear as the bond grows in intensity.

During this investigation or during other periods of particular distress in therapy, the survivor's ability to heal and grow may be restricted by overwhelming emotions. When this happens, the survivor may fail to benefit from the therapy, due to her "disabled" state. In this case, the therapist and survivor must work together to empower and "enable" the survivor so that the healing process can continue. Sometimes, a therapist will suggest that the survivor be evaluated by a psychiatrist for possible psychotropic medication of the symptoms (such as anxiety, panic, dread, and depression). If the psychiatrist agrees with the assessment of the therapist, he/she may prescribe medication for use by the survivor. Most medications are taken consistently, once or twice per day, though a few medications are taken in response to specific increases in symptoms. For instance, when a wave of panic hits, a survivor may use a single tablet to reduce those feelings, while in another situation, a survivor whose depression has become increasingly worse during "talk therapy" may use a daily medication to help reduce her symptoms.

Medication is generally used to get the survivor "over the hump." It is rarely prescribed for more than twelve to eighteen months, as many medications are addictive or have side effects. The therapist who suggests temporary psychotropic treatment must also teach the survivor alternative ways to cope with overwhelming feelings, so that the survivor can begin to take control of her own life. Often therapists will instruct survivors on the use of relaxation exercises, positive self-talk, or "stop-thought" techniques. Whichever skills selected by the therapist, the survivor must learn over time to rely on her own positive, healing behavior, rather than formal medical or therapeutic treatment.

Sexual

"Is there sex after sex abuse?"

As is outlined in Chapter 4, there are many impacts of sexual abuse on the survivor's sensuality and sexuality. While the couple's sex life may be "fine" prior to treatment for sexual abuse issues, this may change over time. Once the issues are opened up, many survivors shut down their sexuality and may even become averse to sexual interaction for a period of time. Often partners wonder if the sexuality of the couple will ever be healed, especially if the survivor is unable to engage in any sexual behavior. As long as the survivor continues to participate in the healing process, a healthy sexuality will develop. The efforts of the survivor and his or her partner are what determine the rate and range of sexual healing.

> *Since my wife entered therapy for her abuse issues, our sex life has disappeared completely. What's up with this? Are we ever going to have sex again?*

While most survivors do experience a reduction or temporary cessation of their sexual desire while exploring their abuse issues, sexuality is generally restored as issues are defused and memories and feelings are integrated. The healing of sexuality generally occurs after the survivor has managed her feelings of shame, despair, hopelessness, loss, and anger. Sexuality is an expression of power and vulnerability, and the survivor must regain and repossess strength previously invested in maintaining the silence of sexual abuse.

> *My girlfriend has trouble having an orgasm. Is there anything we can do differently to make it happen? I like to be very creative sexually, but my partner insists on a rigid sexual routine. Is there any hope of her relaxing and learning to enjoy variety?*

In order for the survivor to heal her sexuality, she must be ready to forgive and accept her body as a source of pride and pleasure. This process rarely begins before the survivor has spent time in psychotherapy, mourning her losses and confronting her demons. When she is able to integrate her sexual abuse as part of her life story minus the overwhelming emotions that have been attached to memories in the past, she is ready to incorporate her body as a productive and pleasure-giving vehicle.

The degree to which a survivor heals her sexuality depends on many factors. The degree to which she was abused (e.g. chronic rape versus single occurrence fondling), the kinds of abuse she endured (as well as the physical sites which were abused), and the beliefs she has about sexuality all impact her ability to develop a healthy sexuality. A survivor who has been repeatedly sodomized by her abuser may never want to engage in anal intercourse, though she may enjoy vaginal intercourse and oral sex. Likewise, a survivor whose breasts were often pinched by her abuser may not be stimulated by caresses on her breasts, but may be enthusiastic about having her partner stroke, lick and enter her vagina.

The extent to which the survivor is able to heal determines the range of sexual behaviors in which the survivor will be able to engage. Should the survivor participate in the healing process only to the level which enables her to enjoy basic sexual interaction, it is unlikely that she will be comfortable with a large variety of sexual behaviors. If the couple enjoys a simple sex life, then the survivor need not go beyond this point. If the survivor's goal is to feel comfortable in any sexual situation (I think there are probably very few non-survivors who have met this goal!), then she will probably have to expend a great deal of energy healing her sexuality and sensuality. Whether the survivor can achieve orgasm while engaging in these sexual behaviors depends on additional factors.

Alice's story in Chapter 4 identified some of the issues which effect the survivors ability to orgasm. For most individuals, orgasm leaves them momentarily incapacitated, or out of control. For the survivor, this may be terrifying. Given this, she may need to work her way up to orgasm. If the survivor can find a safe place in her home where she can masturbate, she may be able to learn to orgasm alone. If she is unable to orgasm with private, manual stimulation, she may want to use a sexual aid such as a vibrator, which stimulates the genitals vigorously and may facilitate orgasm.

When the survivor is able to achieve orgasm by herself, she may opt to work toward orgasm with her partner. During the initial efforts with her partner, the survivor may want to be sexual, without the goal of orgasm, remaining relaxed at all times. When she is able to maintain sexual stimulation and relaxation concurrently, she can begin to focus on achieving orgasm. The survivor can use positive self-talk and erotica to maintain relaxation and positive body images, but may also need the support of her partner. Orgasm occurs when the couple is able to engage in consenting sexual activity, in which both partners are treated equally and with respect. Mutual trust and the maintenance of secure, positive feelings enable the survivor to relax and enjoy. For further information on healing sexuality and enhancing sexual interaction, refer to the resources guide in Chapter 10.

> *Any time I "talk dirty" to my girlfriend when we're having sex, she freezes up and spaces out? What's this about?*

Many perpetrators verbally and emotionally abuse their victims, as well as sexually abuse them. Children who do not have the experience or capabilities to understand the sexually stimulating aspects of erotic talk experience this as frightening and intimidating (as well as confusing).

When a survivor enters a sexual relationship and her partner uses erotic language, it is likely that the survivor will associate the language with her abuse. If she has been working through these issues, she may be able to repress old memories and move on to sexual enjoyment. More than likely, the survivor's sexual desire will diminish immediately. If she is able to discuss this with her partner, and he/she is willing to try alternative sexual behaviors, she may be able to resume her sexual activity and experience pleasure. If she feels incapacitated, or is unable to stop the interaction to talk with her partner, she may withdraw through dissociation. In other words, if the survivor is emotionally overwhelmed and unable to physically withdraw from her source of distress, she may mentally retreat. When the survivor spaces out or splits, the partner will probably recognize the survivor's failure to connect with him/her. It may seem as if the survivor is somewhere else, which in essence, she is (where depends on the survivor's symbols and images of safety). If this should happen, it is important that the partner stop the activity that the couple is engaged in and ask the survivor to talk about what is happening. The partner must push aside his/her own sexual desire in order to respect the emotional needs of the survivor, with the knowledge that sexual activity will resume sometime in the future.

> *I've noticed a change in my partner in recent months: when we have sex, he wants me to be aggressive, even rough with him. I know what happened to him, and I'm afraid that if I agree to some of the things he asks for, I'll become just like his abuser. Should I go ahead, or not?*

Sexual variety is wonderful, and playing out fantasies can be fun for both survivor and partner. When a survivor is repeating behaviors from the past, especially those that have been dangerous or caused him physical or emotional harm, it is important that the survivor really analyze his desires before fulfilling them. If the survivor is unwilling to do so and encourages his partner to cause him physical pain, it is up to the partner to limit the couple's sexual activities.

Repeating sexually abusive behaviors in order to master or gain control over them is a fairly common occurrence among survivors. Unless the survivor selects a supportive partner who can guide the survivor through the process step by step without causing further emotional damage, these behaviors can do more harm than good. Engaging in violent sex can leave the sexual abuse survivor with a negative sense of self and a limited sense of esteem or self-worth.

Emotional
"How many ups balance a down?"

It is often difficult for the survivor to maintain balance in his or her life, especially while exploring abuse issues. The survivor sheds many tears and shouts hundreds of curses in order to find just one smile during some months. And at other times, the survivor feels really good about him- or herself, even when relating painful memories. Not only is this wave-like motion of healing difficult for the survivor to manage, but it is hard for the partner to recognize that these ups and downs will flatten out with time and emotional growth.

> *My girlfriend says she has a great deal of trouble completely trusting me, yet I feel like she trusts me a lot. She told me about the abuse, and we have a close relationship, but somehow she feels like she still doesn't trust me. How do I interpret this and what can I do?*

Trust is very subjective. For the survivor, betrayal of trust has pervaded her life. When she was vulnerable and trusted as a child, someone came along and betrayed that trust and abused her. Whether or not they knew that the abuse was occurring, the survivor may have experienced her parents as non-protective. They, too, betrayed her trust. Others who failed to assist her or recognize her pain are experienced as untrustworthy. The survivor must overcome great resentment, shame and pain before she is even ready to trust again.

When she is willing to invest her trust in another human being, the survivor may test the individual for an extensive period of time, as she tries to determine whether they will betray her. Although the partner may interpret certain behaviors as reflection of trust, the survivor may still be testing her partner out. The trust develops after many tests, and over much time, and as a result of empathy, support, and love.

> *It seems to me that my girlfriend is very high strung. Things are often much more emotional than they need to be and she often tries to run away from me, saying that she wishes I didn't love her. When she finally calms down, she tells me that she's afraid that I'll leave her, even though I have no intention of doing so. How do I deal with this?*

There are many reasons why emotions may run high in the survivor, but a common reason is lack of emotional practice. Most survivors learn early on that feelings make a personal vulnerable. Because the perpetrator has already made the survivor vulnerable through the abuse, the survivor is not likely to intentionally increase her feelings of vulnerability. She learns to restrict her range of emotions, and remain cool and aloof. She becomes independent and self-sufficient over time, as she recognizes that interactions can be dangerous as they elicit overwhelming and often untapped emotions. Unfortunately, when the survivor meets a partner with whom she would like to interact on an intimate level, she finds herself confused and unpracticed in matters of the heart.

As the survivor learns to open herself to the impact and support of her partner, she may find that more of her protective wall tumbles than she originally desired or intended. She may be left feeling quite vulnerable and exposed and may then be even more sensitive to emotions that are elicited between her and her partner. The shame she has experienced since the onset of the abuse may also resurface with the rest of her emotions, causing her to fear rejection by her partner. While she may desire the relationship, it is associated with all of the emotional changes she has undergone. While she was independent and alone, the survivor was able to cap her emotions and remain distanced from her fears. When she is particularly overwhelmed, she is likely to want to reject the relationship and all changes which accompanied its development. Offering consistent support to the survivor and repeating your commitment to the relationship may enable her to feel more comfortable about the numerous changes she is undergoing.

Is there a good or bad way to deal with the frequent mood swings that my partner has?

Some mood swings arise as a result of the survivor's lack of practice with his/her emotions. Other mood swings reflect a chemical imbalance which can be treated with psychotropic medication. Encourage your partner to speak with his/her therapist about the source of these emotional fluctuations. If the mood swings cycle consistently and are associated with alternating periods of depression and mania (e.g. racing thoughts, increased activities, decreased need for sleep, etc.), then it is possible that medication may enable your partner to remain on a more even keel. If the mood swings are associated with certain people, behavior, or places, it is possible that the survivor is being triggered, or reminded in idiosyncratic ways of his/her abuse issues. If this is the case, then it is important that the survivor learn to identify his/her triggers, and learn to soothe or parent him- or herself in response to these stimuli.

In addition to supporting the survivor's work in therapy, it is important that the partner recognize the triggers and avoid presenting them at all costs. If you are unable to avoid some trigger situations, offer support and strength to the survivor as he/she confronts the emotions which are generated in response to the trigger. If the survivor is overwhelmed by the trigger and your presence increases his/her anxiety, fear or rage, offer to leave the survivor alone for a while, or to provide the survivor with a symbol or image of safety and security.

> *I feel caught in a catch 22 sometimes when I know my wife wants me to be honest with her but I also know that she gets very emotional, so sometimes I let things pass and then in the end, they erupt. Either way, a problem is vented. Should I just be honest all the time?*

Because survivors tend to be hypervigilant or super-sensitive, they can often spot a lie a mile away. If you are not truthful with your partner, she will resent you, even if you see your lies as "protective." A survivor has endured incredible trauma and lived to tell her story. Dealing with painful information or a difficult situation is not going to kill her. Her reaction may be uncomfortable for both of you but will diffuse over time, but if she must confront a lie, she is likely to feel betrayed and disrespected. In the end, it is likely to require less energy of the couple to cope with the truth.

Psychological
"Can an old dog learn new tricks?"

Survivors can learn new ideas and coping skills at any age and so can you! No matter how long ago the abuse occurred, the survivor can stop using unhealthy coping mechanisms and begin to live a more satisfying life—if he/she wants to. Changing one's lifestyle takes a lot of time, energy, and commitment. The survivor who learns to live differently cannot alter who he/she is, but can change how he or she is accomplishing goals in his/her life. Sexual abuse transforms the fabric of the survivor's life. The survivor can take control and change the color of the thread or alter the pattern of the weave, but the origination of the fabric will always remain the same.

> *My wife is just starting to remember abuse that happened a long time ago. What do I do? Are there resources out there for her? How about for me?*

When survivors "pop" their memories, major shifts occur. During the emergent phase, it is important to provide the survivor with constant emotional support and nurturing. She may want to talk at odd times of the day or night, may need her partner to soothe and calm her when she experiences nightmares or flashbacks, but primarily will need the love and comfort of a partner who can help her diminish her feelings of fear and shame.

It is also important that the survivor receive the kind of professional care that she deserves. Some survivors are able to work through their issues in outpatient psychotherapy, but others may need more intensive treatment at the outset, or during times of particular difficulty. Inpatient care is available across the country, with many facilities specializing in the treatment of sexual abuse. Survivors may benefit from short-term crisis care, in crisis houses or "half-way houses," or may need the more extensive treatment available through long-term residential facilities. A large percentage of survivors will seek temporary crisis or emergent care at some point during their treatment for sexual abuse issues.

If the survivor is able to manage her issues in outpatient psychotherapy, it is likely that the therapist will want to see both the survivor and the couple. Often the partner is asked to participate in treatment, not only to assist and support the survivor, but also to attend to the partner's issues and needs. Recognizing sexual abuse and managing the impacts made by this kind of trauma takes every ounce of energy that the couple can muster. Especially if the abuse issues have been repressed for a long period of time, the energy required to uncover and explore these images and memories is considerable.

In addition to outpatient psychotherapy for the survivor, the couple, and the partner if he chooses, there are a number of additional resources available. The couple may be asked to begin reading about sexual abuse or to journal the thoughts and feelings which arise in daily life together. They may be encouraged to view videos or films on sexual abuse and its effects on the survivor, couple and family. The therapist may suggest that the survivor attend group therapy for survivors or Sexual Abuse Anonymous support groups. The partner may even want to get further support for himself in a therapy group for partners. These resources are further summarized in Chapter 10.

> *I know that sexual abuse has had a big impact on my husband. How much of his personality is due to the sexual abuse, and how much just reflects the way he is?*

The personality of the survivor often reflects a combination of genetics, socialization, and the impacts of sexual abuse (nature, nurture, and nihilation). While it would be impossible to lay percentages on these specific components, there are certain factors which may enable the survivor to better understand himself and the development of his personality. Most investigators believe that the personality or "self" is developed during the first few years of life, and that events and experiences following that period only mold the foundation that has already been laid. If the sexual abuse occurred after age five, the impacts of the sexual abuse may change the way that the survivor lives and behaves, but may not necessarily change the core of his personality structure. What we often see of the individual is the way he acts, emotes, and thinks. Some portion of what we observe reflects his internal core, but how much? No one truly has the answer to that question.

Sexual abuse changes the survivor. It changes how he looks at the world, it alters how he perceives himself, and it transforms how he interacts with others in his environment. Thoughts, feelings, and behaviors change in accordance with these other transformations. While treatment for sexual abuse issues may not alter the core personality structure, it will have an impact on perceptions, thoughts, emotions, coping strategies, and behavior.

What can I do to help my girlfriend "relax and enjoy the ride"? She always seems to be in control and I'd like for her to mellow out a little and let me take the reins at times.

Survivors often thrive on control. After being abused, and feeling totally helpless, it is natural for the individual to assume total control over self and to desire to control her interactions with others.

Abuse is generally confusing, unpredictable, and extremely threatening (in addition to traumatic). Once free from the abusive situation, the survivor seeks interactions and situations in which she will not have to experience these emotions again. The survivor may learn to restrict her emotions, especially when in public, so that others are not aware of how she is feeling. If they are blind to her true feelings, these can not be used against her, as her emotions may have been used by her abuser. She may try to control as much of her environment as possible so that there are no surprises with which to contend. She may become hypervigilant so that she has information about everything occurring in her environment, and can avoid feeling confused. She may assume control in order to feel powerful at last.

Given her needs for control and comprehension, the survivor may be unable to share the power with another person. Unfortunately, this does not bode well for a relationship, unless the partner is willing to be submissive and compliant. When these needs for comprehensive control begin to threaten the survivor's support system, it is important that she seek counseling to explore these issues. As the partner is also affected by these factors, it is important that he/she also participate in the therapy.

Most survivors find that they are most comfortable when they can assert control over certain situations, such as sexual interaction. The couple may need to work together to identify specific situations that are especially difficult for the survivor, and in which she can feel powerful. It is also important that the partner feel comfortable in situations in which he/she generally feels anxious or distressed. In the remaining situations, it is important that control be shared. Each partner may also need to identify a few images or thoughts that are soothing, so that if the shared control generates anxiety or other overwhelming emotions, the partners can initiate some relaxation.

Learning to relax and enjoy the ride may take a while, but can be achieved if both partners are willing to work together and provide tolerance, support and nurturing.

> *How come my boyfriend thinks that every bad outcome is his fault, while not acknowledging any of his accomplishments?*

There are many reasons why individuals become self-deprecating or self-critical. One reason that survivors assume blame and focus on their negatives stems from the abuse situation itself. When the child is abused, he feels confused, ashamed, and helpless. Because these feelings are intolerable, he searches for other emotions that cause less pain. Often, children will assume guilt, or responsibility for the abuse in order to feel less helpless. The logic is nonsensical, but allows the child to reduce some of the feelings which he experiences as intolerable. Even after the abuse has been terminated, the child continues to use this coping strategy.

The child begins to experience guilt rather than helplessness, and, because he "caused the abuse to happen," he begins to perceive himself as bad and shameful. He may believe then, that he deserved the abuse, and that he deserves other bad things that happen to him (because he sees himself as a bad boy). Even as an adult, the survivor continues to emphasize self-deprecation, criticism and guilt, even when his accomplishments merit self-esteem. As the survivor explores his abuse issues, and learns to forgive himself for being a child, and can finally allow the perpetrator to take responsibility for the abuse, the survivor may begin to recognize his inner goodness and value. Then, and only then, will the survivor begin to recognize his accomplishments and experience pride.

Are the hallucinations experienced during a "flashback" like those of fever or drug hallucinations?

I am not aware of any medical research that has been conducted to date on the flashbacks of survivors. Clinical research indicates that there is one major difference between flashbacks and hallucinations: during flashbacks, consciousness is generally not altered. Conversely, during some fever-induced hallucinations and drug "trips," the individual may actually lose consciousness and experience his dreams and mental images as "real." In both hallucinatory and flashback experiences, the individual apparently enters a parallel perceptual bank, filled with images from memory or fantasy which are then experienced as current reality. Lenore shares her experiences below:

> *It is usually the same: we are close to one another, perhaps lying in the darkness, when the tall shadow appears. The darkness fills the room, save a small crack of light which falls over his shoulder. As he approaches, the room shifts: my pink sheets fade and a tiny flower pattern spreads across the old white sheets. My window has moved from one wall to the other. The comforting body beside me has vanished and I am alone once again to deal with this monster. It is not until the familiar shadow has nearly encompassed me and I can smell the alcohol on his breath before Ed's voice booms inside my head, "Lenore, where are you? Lenore are you OK?" I can not see him, I can only see this monster from my past, but I know that Ed is the light at the end of my tunnel, and I must move steadily forward, through the shadows to reach him and my own mental sanctuary.*

While those who "trip" must wait for the drugs to be processed and expelled by the body in order for the hallucinations to stop, and those with fevers must await the break of the fever, survivors must actively fight the images and feelings of the flashback. In order to return to normalcy, the survivor must use his or her symbols of the present to reconnect to reality. When a supportive partner is available, the partner can act as a safe guide back to the present. It is important to use caution: some survivors perceive and experience others in their environments as individuals from the past. Partners must tread lightly and offer support and security. Should the survivor experience the partner as threatening, it is important that the partner move away from the survivor, but continue to offer threads of reality, and validations of comfort and safety.

Is it easier to cope with sexual abuse issues when the perpetrator is dead or in prison?

Memories of past sexual abuse often do not pop until the perpetrator is incapacitated, incarcerated or dead. Images return from repression when it is safe for the survivor to remember. Memories may return when the individual has developed a supportive network or a nurturing intimate relationship. They may arise as the survivor's self-esteem increases, or when major life goals have been accomplished. When the survivor is able to manage the memories and images, they will resurface.

Once sexual abuse memories have been reintegrated into the conscious state, the survivor must decide how to proceed. Most enter therapy at some point. Many process these old images in writing or art. As the survivor begins to accept the reality of what has occurred, he/she may want to confront her abuser and those who failed to protect her from the trauma. If the perpetrator is dead, the survivor may feel "cheated," as she is then unable to confront the abuser directly. This does not prohibit her from making a confrontation. It simply means that she cannot experience the reaction of the perpetrator when confronted.

If the perpetrator has been incarcerated for sexual abuse and is receiving treatment for these issues in prison, the survivor may actually be invited to participate. Often, perpetrators in specialized programs are encouraged to elicit confrontations from those they abused, so that they can begin to recognize the consequences of their actions. Perpetrators may simply listen, or may offer apologies, sometimes even in the form of financial restitution (often used to pay the survivor's therapy costs).

If the perpetrator has been incarcerated for another reason, the survivor must decide whether or not to confront him/her. While some survivors gain a sense of safety and security from a perpetrator's imprisonment (for any reason), others actually experience greater fear. A perpetrator who has been punished for additional crimes may be experienced as even more threatening, inhibiting the survivor's confrontation.

Spiritual
"Why hast Thou forsaken me?"

Survivors often experience spiritual confusion as they explore their sexual abuse issues. They wonder, "Why me?" searching for answer which is consistent with their spiritual beliefs. Survivors are often unable to find such an answer, because the selection of victims and the experience of violation is randomly determined. Sexual abuse happens because a perpetrator chooses to act out. The child is selected to fill the perpetrator's needs. The choice of a particular child reflects the perpetrator's fantasies and needs for convenience. No child is responsible for the sexual abuse committed by a perpetrator.

Will my partner ever be able to truly believe in
God again after enduring such horrible abuse?

Many survivors are unable to manage the discrepancies experienced between religious faith and sexual abuse. These survivors remain separate from formal religious orders and form their own spiritual beliefs. Others, whose support networks may be limited, need the support of the Church to facilitate their survival. If the survivor's "original" Church is able to provide support without judgment, the survivor's healing may progress rapidly. If the survivor's original Church is critical and holds the survivor responsible (in any way) for the sexual abuse, the survivor may need to try alternative sites for worship. Spiritual healing is an important factor in the survivor's recovery, but is often left to the end stages of healing (if sought at all).

Are there some religious faiths which promote healing better than others?

Religion offers a great deal of support, but also presents many complications to the survivor. Faiths which are based on the "God-fearing" concept, tend to focus on the limited capacity of the individual. These religious faiths often suggest that the individual must accomplish a certain set of tasks in order to keep God happy, and in order to "qualify" for entrance into Heaven. Frequently, these faiths require their members to follow a rigid structure including twice or thrice weekly worship, maintaining certain beliefs, and cultivating converts. The belief systems of these religious orders often emphasize sin-induced shame and guilt, two of the most harmful emotions for the survivor to experience (because they validate the negative self-images which have already been generated by the sexual abuse). Since the survivor is attempting to increase acceptance of his/her "self" and reduce feelings of shame and guilt, religious orders which inhibit this process should be avoided. This may mean that survivors who have been raised in certain religious orders may want to try alternative religious orders.

Faiths which emphasize God's love of man and woman, and the inherent goodness of all people may offer the survivor more support. These Churches often focus on retaining members of the congregation through acceptance and adaptation, rather than on cultivating certain types of members. In some areas of the country, community churches are available which offer worship service focusing on universal messages rather than on Biblical interpretations. In other areas, where community churches are not available, the survivor may need to "try out" a host of local Churches to determine which offer the kind of support most accessible to the survivor.

My partner is a devout Christian and firmly believes in "Original Sin," so she thinks that the abuse is all her fault. How can I help her realize that she wasn't responsible?

It is difficult to "undo" the training the survivor receives during the sexual abuse. It may be even more difficult to unravel an individual's religious upbringing in order to promote spiritual healing. Often, when the survivor can attend to the statistics about sexual abuse, she can begin to recognize how widespread and random it really is. If one in every two or three women is sexually abused during her lifetime, and both children and elders are equally demeaned and denigrated, it is unlikely that the survivor can assume personal responsibility for her abuse.

It is important to focus on the responsibility of the perpetrator when exploring sexual abuse issues. The survivor can be responsible for making bad choices and for actions she made, but it is important that she not attempt to take the responsibilities of the perpetrator as her own. Not only does this increase her pain, guilt and shame, but it relieves the perpetrator of the burden he/she must rightfully carry. If the survivor protects the perpetrator from the consequences of his/ her actions (by assuming guilt and blame for the abuse), the perpetrator will continue to abuse children without regard to the consequences of the abuse for them.

When Bad Things Happen to Good People offers a beautiful understanding of this very complex issue.

> *My partner's religious beliefs have prompted her to forgive her family and her abuser. I have a strong faith as well, but I can't see how she can forgive them for what they did. Do all survivors forgive their abusers at some point? Is this healthy?*

Forgiving the self is an important step for the survivor. Forgiving the perpetrator is optional. Some survivors believe that forgiveness enables the survivor to let go of the abuse. Others believe that it is important to maintain some of the pain and anger in order to prohibit the abuse from happening again (to the survivor or to another). Survivors must choose whether or not to forgive their abusers. Should the survivor choose to forgive, it is important that she do so at the appropriate point in her healing: when she has allowed herself to experience her losses, rage, resentment, disappointment, and pain. Only when she has recognized and experienced these emotions can she truly consider whether or not she can let them go. Should she make an effort to forgive prior to the accomplishment of this goal, she will harbor feelings of resentment and anger, and experience guilt and shame for doing so.

> *My partner was victimized by a priest. What kind of counseling should I help him find? Somehow he has to learn that not all representatives of the Church are bad.*

As time goes by, and more survivors tell their stories of abuse, more representatives of the Church are exposed for their abuses. Survivors of sexual abuse by a Church authority (e.g. a minister) experience a very painful confusion about their spirituality and religious upbringing. Not only do they become fearful and suspicious of other ministers and priests, but they continue to harbor resentment and anger at the Church for "leading them to the slaughter." These survivors must actively heal from the damage done to their spiritual selves in addition to surviving the sexual abuse itself.

The survivor who has been abused by a priest or minister will need long-term therapy in order to deal with these issues. Initially, the survivor will probably be more receptive to a secular therapist, who has limited association with the abusive Church. Once, the survivor has begun the healing process, it will be important for the therapist to begin exploring the survivor's feelings of betrayal by the Church. In addition, it may benefit the survivor to meet with a pastoral counselor in order to explore these issues more thoroughly. If the survivor continues to be intimidated by Church representatives, his partner can offer to accompany him, or the secular therapist can invite the pastoral counselor to join them during their regular therapy sessions (after the survivor and therapist have discussed this at length). The survivor may be able to reintegrate the Church into his life with sufficient support and time, or he may choose to remain separate from the institution associated with the abuse.

Relational

"Can love conquer all?" Is it reasonable to ever expect a "normal" relationship where we aren't always talking about and dealing with sexual abuse?

Sexual abuse doesn't ever go away. As the survivor gets further along in his/her healing process, the sexual abuse issues will require less and less energy of the survivor and the couple. During times of major change or transition, though, you can expect that the sexual abuse issues will resurface for a brief period. As the changes are managed and the transitions are completed, the sexual abuse issues will once again fade into the background. While one can not predict the times when the survivor sees his/her abuser in the grocery, or when he/she interacts with a child whose age is the same as when he/she was abused, or when another memory of sexual abuse "pops" loose, you can rest assured that the more the survivor heals, the less time and energy will be spent recovering from these "surprise attacks." As long as both of you actively participate in the healing process, love, joy and laughter can move to the forefront of your lives.

My partner and I are both survivors. Is there any hope for us as a couple?

Dual survivor couples present some unique gifts and challenges to growth and healing. When survivors develop an intimate relationship, they may experience greater understanding of one another than a survivor-non-survivor couple. For this reason, they may also experience greater empathy and compassion for one another. The dual survivor couple may be more prepared to cope with emotional emergencies and flashbacks, because each member has an inherent understanding of the process.

The dual survivor couple also brings with it some unique challenges. When two survivors commit to one another, they must negotiate time and energy for their emergencies, traumas, and reactions. They must alternate the caretaking, the assumption of responsibilities, and the positive parenting.

Should both survivors be emotionally disabled at the same time, it may be difficult for the relationship to survive. Occasionally, survivors in dual survivor couples find themselves jockeying for position, trying to emphasize the extent of their abuse, and minimizing the abuse of their partners in order to become the center of attention. Survivors in these situations may become insensitive as they try to bully their partners into nurturing them, even though the partners may also need support. When both survivors are feeling low, they may feed off one another, each becoming more depressed and hopeless. Should one survivor harm him- or herself, the other emotional health of the other survivor may plummet.

Each couple manages differently. If one member of the couple has spent more time healing from the sexual abuse, he/she may be able to offer support and guidance to his/her partner without being overwhelmed. When this survivor needs support, he/she is more likely to assert his/her needs, and if he/she is unable to meet them in the relationship, it is likely that his/her resource network will be large enough to provide sufficient support. This does not excuse one partner from providing emotional support to the other simply because that partner is further along in the process. It simply means that if the less "able" survivor is not able to function fully as a partner for some reason, the other, more "able" survivor may be able to manage the situation effectively by using his/her support network.

Are sexual abuse survivors more worried about commitment in a relationship than non-survivor partners?

I don't believe that survivors are more worried about commitment in their relationships than non-survivors on the whole. Survivors are probably more sensitive to rejection than others. Because survivors often experience shame and guilt as a result of the abuse, they often perceive themselves as bad or unworthy. They expect others to reject them as soon as it becomes apparent that the survivor is "bad." For this reason, they may wish to gain commitment from their partners, as a pledge to stand by the survivor, even when her faults and negative qualities are uncovered.

Am I always going to have to take care of my partner? Will she ever be able to nurture and emotionally support me?

When the survivor first begins to explore her abuse issues, she requires support from anyone who will offer it. The emerging memories may impair the survivor's ability to care for herself, and the partner may have to help the survivor to achieve basic functions. The partner must provide nurturing, comfort and care, as the survivor searches for a healthy balance between her sexual abuse issues and the rest of her life. This phase may vary in duration, but will likely last for at least a year. As the survivor becomes more able to manage her issues, her strength and ability will reemerge, and her independence will increase. As the survivor becomes better able to manage her issues, it is important that she begin to "put back" into the relationship. The survivor can become an equal partner who can "give" and nurture as much as her non-survivor partner. With adequate therapy and time, the couple can learn to balance their need and support of one another.

Should I ask my partner the details of what happened to her during the abuse?

Most survivors carry a tremendous amount of shame about their sexual abuse. In order to heal, survivors need to integrate their images and memories of their sexual abuse as part of their life tapestries. Breaking the silence and telling their stories allow survivors to reduce shame and bond with others. It is important that this process is at the survivor's own pace. Although each survivor is different, I believe that most survivors would feel nurtured and supported by a partner who cared enough to ask about the details of the abuse. Such curiosity or concern may be interpreted as an indication of total acceptance of the survivor by the partner ("I'll care for you no matter what happened to you").

Prior to eliciting such a disclosure, the partner should ask himself/herself if he/she is capable of tolerating the details. If the partner finds that he/she is unable to manage such a disclosure, it is important that he/she be honest with the survivor. For instance, the partner might say, "I want to provide you with support and show you how much I love and accept you, but I don't think I am prepared to hear all of the details yet." If the partner is willing to hear the disclosure, it is important to respect the story and the feelings of the survivor, and just as important to respect and consider his/her own feelings and needs. For more specific guidelines for managing a disclosure, review Christine Courtois' suggestions in Healing the Incest Wound or the suggestions in Chapter 7 of this book.

Parenting
"Will the circle be unbroken?"

One of the survivor's greatest fears is that he/she will sexually abuse his/her own child, even though the desire to break the cycle of abuse may be strong. The fear is often warranted: research suggests that 50 to 75% of children who are abused or who witness abuse go on to abuse as well. Parent education and training can be an important part of the process for the survivor and his/her partner.

> *For a long time, my partner rejected the idea of having a child, for fear that she would end up abusing the child as her parents abused her. Now, she has begun to look forward to parenthood, and to raising her child in a healthy environment. Will her fears resurface after the child is born?*

Even when parents-to-be believe that they are prepared for the birth of their child, most feel somewhat anxious and overwhelmed following the infant's arrival. Survivors, like non-survivor parents, experience apprehensions and feelings of inadequacy in the time before they "get the hang of things." Survivors may feel tense and uncertain the first time they must change the baby's diaper and clean his or her genitalia. If the survivor has attended community or hospital parent training classes, and receives support for his/her initial efforts, apprehensions quickly fade away as routines are established.

For survivors, the fears associated with the cycle of sexual abuse often arise more intensely when the parent becomes isolated, has few resources, and is unable to cope with stressors that occur. Parents who begin to feel overwhelmed, and question their capabilities may begin to act out with their children, perhaps neglecting the child's needs or even verbally or emotionally abusing the child. Should the parent question his/her own sexuality or experience pedophilic (sexual excitement in response to observing or interacting with a child), then it is even more likely that the parent will sexually abuse the child. While some parents have pedophilic urges, others simply respond to the pubescent changes occurring in the child. These parents tend to be extremely sexist and possessive and see their children as chattel, to be used as the parent so desires. These parents often dominate others and consider all sexually "mature" individuals as objects of pleasure.

When the survivor feels certain that he/she will not abuse the child, but fears that someone else may, the parent may become overly protective and restrict the child's actions. These fears generally become stronger as the child nears the age at which the parent was sexually abused. While the overprotective efforts may reduce the child's chance of being abused, it may increase the child's dependency on the parents, and may inhibit emotional and interpersonal growth.

How will the extra baggage of sexual abuse affect my girlfriend's behavior as a parent?

Sexual abuse survivors often follow two divergent paths: either they become quite rigid and demanding of their children, or they become overly permissive with their children.

Those that emphasize control are often overprotective and fear that their children will be violated as they have been. These parents may recognize their own issues and want to "create" children who can "take care of themselves." This may mean that the child must meet great expectations and achieve numerous goals (such as good grades, excellent performance in sports, and a respectful but commanding interpersonal style).

Those who emphasize permissiveness with their children often lead chaotic and disorganized lifestyles. They may or may not recognize their own sexual abuse issues, but are generally not concerned with the signs and symptoms presented by their children. They require little of their children, and may feel overwhelmed when their children make too many demands on them. These parents have trouble parenting themselves and in times of stress may even coax their children into assuming more responsibility than is healthy for them.

In addition to the common parenting styles often portrayed by survivors, are the fears about protecting their children from the traumas that the parent has survived. These are described in the response above.

Finally, if the parent has begun treatment for his/her sexual abuse issues since the birth of the child, the child may actually observe and experience much of the traumatic impacts that the sexual abuse has had on the parent. The parent may go through rough spots during therapy and may even require hospitalization at some point. Further, while the parent is actively working through his/her sexual abuse issues, he/she may need to require more from his/her co-parent. Should the survivor feel unable to parent the child at any time during the initial stages of the healing process, the co-parent may have to work independently for a time. This early healing period may be experienced by the child as chaotic and up-ending, and may even be upsetting for the child. In order to prevent distress in the child, it is important to help him/her understand as much about the healing process as he/she is able to understand, in a language that is appropriate for his/her age level.

> *I've read a lot about the vicious cycle of abuse and I'm afraid that my husband, who is a survivor, will abuse our children. I'm too ashamed to talk to my husband about these fears. Is there anything I can do to prevent this from happening, or at least to reduce the risk? What are the odds that he will abuse our children?*

Survivors who are receiving treatment are less likely to abuse their own children while in therapy. If they are insightful and experience growth, maturation and the development of alternative coping skills while in therapy, there is an even greater chance that they will not continue the cycle of abuse once their treatment is terminated. While the partner cannot actually prohibit the survivor from abusing his children or someone else's, he or she can help the children become less vulnerable to abuse by the survivor and by others.

Children who participate (to the best of their ability) in the treatment of their parents understand the issues and the potential dangers better than children who are left out of the therapy. Even a child as young as five can understand that there are people who touch children in a way that leaves the child feeling "yucky." They can learn to scream, "Stop!" and to run from these individuals, no matter who the perpetrator is. Additionally, children can learn to speak to their parents and to disclose secrets that make them uncomfortable (these are often secrets about abuse that is happening).

Many school children are taught about "good touch/bad touch" and "stranger danger." If this is not a part of their elementary or kindergarten curriculum, take the task on yourself. Help your children understand about positive sexuality, and about the need to protect themselves from potential violation by staying away from strangers, running from those who intimidate, scare, threaten or "make you feel creepy," and by "telling" when something has happened (no matter how weird or ashamed they may feel).

> *I've noticed that our children have begun to explore each other's bodies. What is normal exploration rather than sibling sexual abuse?*

There is no hard-and-fast rule about what constitutes normal sexual exploration between peers and siblings. There are certain developmental guidelines that may enable the parent to more accurately assess what he/she observes. For instance, prior to the age of three, children are relatively uninterested in other people's bodies, but very much enjoy their own bodies. At approximately age three, children become more interested in the differences between males and females and may develop "crushes" on their parents, relatives or friends of the family (i.e. "When I grow up I'm going to marry my daddy"). Between four and eight, children focus on these differences, and begin to visually explore one another (e.g. "play doctor"). It is normal for children to begin same-sex exploration at this time, and continue until the onset of adolescence. It is unusual for children of opposite sexes to explore each other other's bodies tactually, or with their hands. When children begin to act out sexually or perform adult sexual acts with one another, lines may be crossed, and one or both of the children may suffer from feelings of confusion and violation.

> *We've just discovered that our child has been abused by someone in our neighborhood. What do we do now?*

When a child has been abused, there are a number of details that must be attended to. First, it is important to talk with the child and determine what has happened. If any of the child's orifices has been penetrated with a body part or object, it is important that the child be examined by a physician to assess the damage created by the violation. Because the examination may be uncomfortable and frightening for the child, it should be conducted by a physician who is experienced in working with children who have been abused. If your pediatrician is competent to perform the exam, take your child to him/her. If the pediatrician is not skilled in this kind of exam, he/she may have referrals for a pediatrician who specializes in this area. If your pediatrician is unable to make an appropriate referral, the local Child Advocacy Center or Child Protective Service may be able to recommend a physician. Should these sources also come up empty, call your local hospital and ask where the nearest rape crisis team is located. This group of physicians and clinicians may offer to perform the exam or may refer you to a competent pediatrician.

In order to prevent further abuse to your child or to someone else's, it is necessary to make a report to the Child Protective Services in your community. The number may be listed as Child Abuse Hotline in the front of your phone book. You may wish to file a police report, and/or criminal charges with the District Attorney. Your local law enforcement agency can assist you with this process.

When the child's physical safety has been ensured, you must attend to the child's emotional health. While you can help your child overcome the shame, guilt, fear and helplessness associated with sexual violation, you may need some help. Resources for both the family and the child can enable the family to function better as a unit. The child may be treated by a clinician who specializes in the treatment of sexual abuse.

Parents may want to seek their own counseling with the same therapist or another counselor. Finally, survivors of sexual abuse often benefit from talking with one another. Therapy groups for children can sometimes be difficult to locate, but with the assistance of the local Child Protective Services, Office of Family and Child Services, or mental health center, these resources can be identified.

Family of Origin
"To what length, loyalty?"

When a child or adolescent is sexually abused by a family member, it is often extremely difficult for the survivor to separate him- or herself from the perpetrator, especially if there are hopes for continued family interaction. Because it means identifying their parents, siblings and relatives as perpetrators, incest survivors often remain enmeshed in the abusive environment even at the expense of their own mental health.

> *A strange relationship has developed between my partner and her abusive mother and I believe it is detrimental to her healing. What can I do to help?*

Incest survivors often resist separating from their abusive parents because it entails accepting that the parents have treated them inhumanely. It means that the survivor must admit to the reality of the abuse, and let go of the wish to have an ideal family where members treat each other with respect. Separation and independence force the survivor to face the dysfunctional or "sick" dynamics at work in the family unit and to recognize the imperfections of her parents. Because children desire unity and comfort, they are often resistant to separating from their parents, even if the parents have abused them.

If the survivor is willing to separate and explore the incest issues with a therapist, the partner can provide emotional support for the process. If the survivor finds herself constantly returning to the abusive environment, she may want to contract with the partner to help monitor these behaviors. If the partner is returning to a home and is being abused again, you may want to take her for crisis management or inpatient treatment to ensure her safety. If she is not currently being abused, there is little you can do to prevent the survivor from interacting with others, even parents who have been abusive in the past. Provide love and support, and assist the survivor to face the truths of the past and present.

> *My husband still visits his grandfather in the nursing home where he resides now. This man abused him for years, and yet, my husband remains loyal to this old man. Is there something wrong with my husband, or what?*

Abuse survivors are loyal to their perpetrators for many reasons. Survivors who have not really explored their abuse issues in therapy may maintain denial about the abuse, interpreting it as "love." Often perpetrators tell their child victims that sexual behaviors are how people show their love to one another. Between adults, this is an accurate statement, but it is not an accurate description for behaviors which occur between children and adults. When a survivor has grown up with these messages, it may be difficult for him to let go of these ideas and replace them with painful realities. Additionally, if a survivor assumes any responsibility for the abuse, he may not see a connection between his shame and his continued interaction with the perpetrator.

Other survivors remain loyal to their perpetrators in order to be included in settlements and wills. These survivors look forward to the revenge of financial retribution upon the perpetrator's death.

> *After my girlfriend told me about how her stepfather had abused her, I felt so sick and angry. I just wanted to take down my shotgun and blow the guy away. I didn't do it, but I still feel like killing the guy for what he did. What do I do?*

Frequently, when a survivor makes a disclosure to her partner, the partner is overwhelmed by the information. Often, partners feel enraged, disgusted, nauseous, and anxious, and may become homicidal or suicidal. If the partner continues to feel overwhelmed or distressed after a few days, it is important that the partner seek some professional assistance. If the survivor is in therapy, her therapist may offer to see the partner, or may make a referral.

While many partners feel like acting on their desires to threaten, harm or kill the perpetrator, it is important that the partner not take away control from the survivor. It is vital that the survivor control the confrontations with the perpetrator, otherwise she may begin to feel violated and disrespected by the partner. This does not mean that the partner should not express his/her feelings about the disclosure or about his/her responses to the disclosure. If the survivor is unable or unwilling to hear her partner's feedback or response, then it is important that the partner seek therapy for him- or herself.

> *After years of abuse by my own father, I ran away. On the road, I met my girlfriend, Lisa, who had recently run away from her mother, who had been sexually abusing her since she was a kid. Lisa told me that she has two little sisters that are still there with her mother and we're both worried about their safety. Is there anything we can do? I can't even face my own father, so I don't know if I'm strong enough to deal with someone else's abuser.*

In cases where one child has been sexually abused, and the perpetrator has access to other children, it is essential that the additional children be protected. While Child Protective Services is often overburdened and unable to investigate every report that it receives, the representatives may be able to help. If there is an outstanding report on the perpetrator, it is more likely that an investigation will be conducted. In addition to filing a report with Child Protective Services, you can call the law enforcement agency in the area where the perpetrator resides and file a formal complaint.

If the survivor is unwilling to confront the perpetrator in person or would be in physical danger by doing she may have to make more indirect efforts to protect the safety of her siblings. If the other children attend school, the survivor may express her concerns to the principal and/or guidance or school counselors at the children's school. If there are supportive relatives or friends of the family who can intervene, contact these people. If the survivor is alone and homeless, she can seek shelter and assistance from the local mission, shelter, or Battered Women's Center. While she may wish to protect her siblings, the survivor cannot help unless she has maintained emotional and physical strength and has attained some legal or relational support. If the survivor is an adult, she can even petition to become the legal guardian for her siblings, but in order to achieve this, the survivor must be able to emotionally and financially support the siblings.

> *The man who abused my wife as a child was a friend of her parents. My wife feels that her parents betrayed her by "leading her to slaughter." What are the chances that my wife will ever work things out with her parents?*

During the healing process, most survivors experience intense anger toward their parents for failing to protect the survivor. This is a normal phase of healing which should not be inhibited. It is important that the survivor be able to vent her feelings with her therapist, partner and/or parents in order to let go of the responsibility she has taken for the abuse. While her parents may not have been directly responsible for the abuse, their friendship with the perpetrator (especially if it was maintained after the onset of the abuse) is associated with the pain and violation that the survivor experienced. For this reason, the survivor benefits from exploring these associations and expressing her feelings about these connections. While survivors may experience rage and resentment toward their parents, if parents are able to attend to these feelings and express their concern and acceptance of the survivor and her pain, the survivor is likely to work toward reintegrating her parents into her life. If parents are critical of the healing process, are defensive, or deny any part of the survivor's story, it is less likely that the survivor will seek to repair the damaged bonds with her unsupportive parents.

Chapter 9
Putting It All Together

Sexual abuse survival is forever. That doesn't mean the survivor will be depressed and angry for the remainder of your relationship with him or her, and it need not mean that the two of you are always working as hard as you're working now. It means that, during times of stress, the relationship must be strong in order to withstand the emotional upheavals of survivor and partner alike.

How can you improve the endurance and strength of your relationship? You've made an effort to begin to understand your partner and the impacts of sexual abuse on him or her, and have even tried to better understand your response to your partner. Now, comes the real challenge: to move forward and begin to make some changes in the way that you function in your relationship. The risks you begin to take may be small at first, but soon, you will see that alternative coping strategies can benefit both of you. This chapter provides the couple with a few helpful hints for developing a healthier and happier relationship.

Communication

As you may remember from Chapter 5, communication is one of the most important components of any healthy relationship. And when you are intimately involved with a survivor, assertive communication becomes even more vital.

Survivors are trained to keep secrets and are told directly or indirectly, "Don't tell!." Even though others may encourage the survivor to speak freely, it is unlikely that he/she will, given the threatening messages that are often used to keep survivors quiet. Given sufficient encouragement and modeling, the survivor can learn to share and express his/her feelings more openly.

In order to keep the lines of communication open with your partner, you may have to make an extra effort to initiate and maintain assertive communication. Offer your opinions, express your feelings, and share your insights (about your own experiences and behaviors) with your partner. Remember that assertiveness requires that you speak honestly, articulately, and respectfully. You must recognize and state your needs and wishes, but you must also be considerate of your partner's feelings. Don't beat around the bush in order not to hurt your partner's feelings, but respect his/her right to feel any way he/she wants to in response to your statements and assertions.

In addition to asserting your needs and desires, it may be helpful for you to make specific requests of your partner as he/she is learning to behave assertively. For instance, you may first want to model the behavior (e.g. by expressing your feelings to your partner). Then, you may want to ask your partner, "How do you feel about (e.g.) my uncle Tony's alcoholism?" This allows your partner to respond to a specific question, and requires very little risk of him or her. As your partner becomes more accustomed to the process, ask broader questions and provide more opportunities for discussion. Soon, you may want to ask the survivor to make disclosures or tell stories about his or her lifetime. If the survivor has not yet told his/her story of abuse, you can provide the opportunity for this as well. As more information is shared between the two of you, you may be able to relax and allow the survivor to take greater control of your interactions. The survivor will ultimately become spontaneous with his/her disclosures and assert his/her needs and wishes with little extra prompting.

Partner Planning

Even when both partners feel capable of asserting their rights and needs, they may not get the chance to interact unless time is put aside for the communication of feelings and ideas. Partner Planning is a process which allows the couple to make time for the basics, and also promotes greater intimacy within the relationship.

If you talk with anyone who lives with a partner, parent, or roommate, he/she will tell you about the complexities of living with another human being (sometimes, you can hardly get them to stop telling you about this!). Just because you are committed to your partner does not guarantee that it will be easy for you to live together. Each person brings emotional baggage and a unique lifestyle to the relationship. In order to manage the similarities and differences between the two of you, you must get to know one another, behave assertively, and take responsibility for your own actions. But to do all of these things, you must take time to talk!

Most couples find that they need to sit down together at least once a week in order to discuss finances, children, career transitions and hassles, major stressors, and emotional fluctuations. When you are involved with a survivor, there may be additions to that list, such as flashbacks, memories, therapy session reviews, personal insights, needs for nurturing, and relationship dynamics. The list is unique for each couple and may be written down to help focus the couple during a Planning session. Sometimes, partners experience relief when they can check off issues or topics as they are reviewed or discussed ("Look how much we've done today!").

A normal Partner Planning session lasts between two and three hours, but can be as long as you need. The session should be held in an environment free of distraction and interruption (including food and sex). The structure of your Planning time is up to you: each partner may want to review the week's ups and downs prior to discussing finances or future plans. Or, you may benefit from addressing the objective issues before discussing feelings and insights. Most importantly, each partner should have an equal opportunity to speak and be heard.

Partner Planning should occur consistently each week (or several times a week if helpful). While you can vary the meeting place if you wish, I would encourage you to keep the time of day stable. Do not attempt to pack activities around the Partner Planning session, as this may cause partners to feel rushed in their reviews and disclosures. Most couples find that Partner Planning increases trust and intimacy in the relationship, but may be somewhat stressful at first.

Partner Planning allows the partners to function as a couple, independent of sex, eating and sleeping. It promotes communication and togetherness, and provides a discrete structure for the interaction. It requires that each partner be assertive and open, and provides an arena for the discussion of thoughts, feelings, and experiences that might otherwise fall through the relational cracks.

Fun Time

In addition to assertive communication, and Partner Planning, the couple needs to have time to play together. As you have read, survivors often feel uncomfortable playing, and may even tell you that they don't know how to play. Survivors experience an overwhelming helplessness when they are abused, and often focus their entire lives on regaining control. Unfortunately, the need to control often prohibits the survivor from relaxing and enjoying life. Survivors may fear that if they let down their guard even a bit, others will take advantage of their vulnerability. They maintain a strict composure and rarely just play.

In addition to the restrictions which survivors may impose on themselves regarding play, they may have been prohibited from playing as children. In incestuous families, child victims are frequently parentified and forced to assume many various adult responsibilities including sexual interaction. If the child is allowed to remain childlike in his/her play, the image may inhibit the perpetrator from sexually abusing his/her child. The perpetrator may prohibit the child from play in efforts to keep the child sexualized and parentified.

Finally, children who are severely abused often isolate themselves from other children in order to hide cuts, bruises, bleeding, and deformities. Additionally, children who are raped often sustain serious physical injury during the process, which may inhibit their range of motion, or ability to walk, run, climb, pump a swing, slide, or jump rope. If the child is abused frequently, he/she could be incapacitated during the developmental years during which play is learned and practiced.

In order for a survivor to play, it may be necessary for his/her partner to teach him/her how to play. If the partner is also inexperienced in this domain, consult your local child, daycare worker or kindergarten teacher.

Exercise #44: "The activities list"

With your partner, make a list of all the fun things that you can think of that the two of you may have missed during childhood. Include activities such as coloring, blowing bubbles, flying a kite, going on a water slide, playing tag, and camping in the woods. Update the list as often as necessary, with ideas and activities offered by all those with whom you interact.

Take time each week to choose an activity from the list and play together! While I am certain that no one can ever tire of childlike play, if you find yourself getting bored with simplicity, be more creative and generate ideas for more advanced play (such as cycling trips, walks in the wilderness, and making crafts together)!

Some forms of play require practice in order for the individual to relax. For instance, when you first learn to swing, gaining height may be frightening, although, over time, achieving great heights may become a goal. For survivors, learning to let go, relax the control, and take comfort in play may take time. Additionally, since survivors generally associate childhood with pain, you may face some resistance in the beginning. If you continue to encourage one another to let loose and be silly, ultimately, the survivor will stop feeling helpless and small, and will begin to recognize him- or herself as a playful adult.

Sexual Healing

As you read in Chapter 4, there are many impacts which sexual abuse has on the survivor's sensuality and sexuality. Additionally, the historical sexual abuse affects the partner's sexuality, as he/she interacts with the survivor. It is important that the lover and survivor work together to heal the survivor's sexuality.

It is vital that the survivor heal at his/her own pace. Initially, the survivor must work alone, to gain feelings of safety in order to explore his/her body visually and tactually. As the survivor becomes more comfortable with self-exploration and masturbation, it is likely that he/she will want to explore his/her partner.

While sexual intercourse may not be forthcoming for a while, the lover and survivor can engage in array of sexual activities which do not require penetration. Initially, it is important that the couple avoid behaviors that have been associated with the original abuse. Over time, the survivor and his/her partner may choose to "defuse" behaviors which have been previously associated with sexual abuse. Suzanne comments on her efforts:

It took Ron and I a long time to get to the point where we wanted to "branch out." We had found a set of behaviors that I was OK with, and we resisted going further. After a while, we actually got a little bored and wanted to remove some of the restrictions on our sexual creativity. During my abuse, I had been fondled, exploited, and vaginally and anally raped. I had overcome my repulsion of vaginal penetration when I got my period, because I had to learn how to insert tampons. The behavior just became more and more routine after that. I had never been able to confront my fear of anal penetration. I still had an absolute repulsion of anal sex, but I didn't want to hate this area of my body any longer. At first, I followed the therapist's instructions to explore my body during my bath. I felt so ashamed the first time I touched my anus, but after a while, I actually learned that it was a very sensitive area of my body that I could gain pleasure from. It took a really long time for me to let Ron touch me there, but when he did, I didn't have to fear. He was gentle and supportive, and held me close while we kissed and explored.

In order to increase the survivor's safety and capacity for sexual interaction, it is important to set aside time for sexual healing. If you have children, take time together when the children are with a sitter, even if it means checking into a hotel! Meet for a rendezvous while the children are at school, or make special time for one another after the children are asleep.

Discuss your needs with one another, and try to find a time and place which is comfortable for both of you. Some survivors do not feel safe indoors, and associate the bedroom and bathroom with abuse. If this is the case, the survivor may feel more comfortable outdoors or in a different environment (such as a hotel). As long as both partners are willing, sexual interludes can occur in the woods, at the beach, or in a car, as long as the environment is safe, free of distraction and interruption, and legal (so that no park ranger comes tapping on your window when you're about to orgasm!). Take the time and energy to relax explore and enjoy one another, so that sexuality can become positive, healthy and fun. Remember, healing takes time.

Final Notes

Healing from sexual abuse takes time, strength, endurance and patience. It also requires that both partners be empathic, considerate, and sensitive to one another's thoughts, feelings, needs and desires. While you may feel like you can't yet see the light at the end of the healing tunnel, stick with it! If you and your partner work together, you can move mountains. The survivor has already proven that he/she has the capacity to endure tremendous pain, and overcome great obstacles. If you are willing to try, the two of you can develop a relationship that meets the challenges set forth by history and current reality.

No one can do it alone. Couples need to use as many resources as they can put their hands on. If a supportive family or friends are available, take them up on their offers of support and distraction. Sometimes, it helps just to have someone with whom to cry or laugh. At other times, you need an objective opinion that you can't find within the relationship. Even if it feels unfamiliar or strange to you, learn to reach out and accept assistance.

Use professional supports as you are able. Seek support from counselors, support and therapy groups, medication and hospitalization if necessary, and 12-step groups (like AA, NA, SAA, ISA, EA and OA) if appropriate. Read everything you can get your hands on dealing with sexual abuse, relationships, and intimacy. If you're not a reader, look for audio and video tapes on these topics.

Listen to others and ask about the interventions and alternative therapies that they've tried. Invest yourself in healing and you will.

Because it is often difficult to know where to turn, I have provided some useful resources in Chapter 10. While the list is far from comprehensive, it offers a place to start. You've already made a tremendous effort. Good luck with your future endeavors!

Chapter 10
Getting Help!

While research in the field of sexual abuse is still unfolding, there are many resources which you may find useful. There are books and guides written for partners, books directed at survivors themselves (which can be informative and helpful for partners as well), newsletters, journals, audio tapes, videotapes, support groups, advocacy councils and inpatient treatment centers. There are even legal resources for survivors who want to prosecute their perpetrators, and treatment centers for incarcerated offenders and those who want help but have yet to be prosecuted. Review the titles, names, and places, and see if there is something that interests you.

Books written especially for partners
As new books are being published every month, the list below may not be comprehensive. It offers a place to start. While you're at the library or book store, spend some time scanning the titles on the shelves. You might find even newer titles that catch your eye.

Davis, Laura (1991). *Allies in Healing*. New York: Harper Perennial.

Engel, Beverly. (1993). *Partners in Recovery*. New York: Fawcett Columbine, 1993.

Gil, Eliana. (1991). *Outgrowing the Pain Together: A Book for Partners and Spouses of Adults Abused as Children*. New York: Dell Bantam Doubleday.

Graber, Ken. (1991). *Ghosts in the Bedroom: A Guide for Partners of Incest Survivors*. Deerfield Beach, FL.: Health Communications.

Hansen, Paul. (1991). *Survivors and Partners: Healing the Relationships of Adult Survivors of Child Sexual Abuse*. Self published. For a copy, send $11.00 to: Paul Hansen, 7548 Cresthill Drive, Longmont, Colorado, 80501

McEnvoy, Alan and Jeff Brookings. (1984). *If She is Raped: A Book for Husbands, Fathers, and Male Friends*. Holmes Beach, FL: Learning Publications.

Books written for survivors
If you'd like more information, or would like to read the material offered to survivors, the list below is filled with books written for and by survivors. If your partner has not yet explored his/her sexual abuse issues, you may want to make a gift of one of the selections below:

Bass, Ellen and Laura Davis. (1988). *The Courage to Heal: A Guide for Women Survivors of Child Sexual Abuse*. New York: Harper & Row.

Bass, Laura and Louise Thornton, eds. (1983). *I Never Told Anyone: Writings by Women Survivors of Child Sexual Abuse*. New York:

Harper & Row.

Bear, Evan, with Peter Dimock. (1988). *Adults Molested as Children: A Survivor's Manual for Women and Men*. Orwell, VT: Safer Society Press. For a copy, send $12.95 to: Shoreham Depot Rd., RR1, Box 24 B, Orwell, VT 05760-9576.

Davis, Laura. (1990). *The Courage to Heal Workbook*. New York: Harper & Row.

Donaforte, Laura. (1982). *I Remembered Myself: The Journal of a Survivor of Childhood Sexual Abuse*. Self-published. For copies, send $7.00 to: P.O. Box 914, Ukiah, CA 95482.

Engel, Beverly. (1989). *The Right to Innocence: Healing the Trauma of Child Sexual Abuse*. Los Angeles, J.P. Tarcher.

Fredrickson, Renée. (1992). *Repressed Memories: A Journey to Recovery from Sexual Abuse*. New York: Simon & Schuster.

Gannon, J. Patrick. (1989). *Soul Survivors: A New Beginning for Adults Abused as Children*. New York: Prentice-Hall.

Hall, Liz and Siobhan Lloyd. (1989). *Surviving Child Sexual Abuse: A Handbook for Helping Women Challenge their Past*. Philadelphia: The Falmer Press.

Sanford, Linda. (1990). *Strong at the Broken Places: Overcoming the Trauma of Childhood Abuse*. New York: Random House.

Books written especially for incest survivors

Blume, E. Sue. (1990). *Secret Survivors: Uncovering Incest and Its Aftereffects on Women*. New York: John Wiley & Sons.

Bronson, Catherine. (1989). *Growing through the Pain. The Incest Survivor's Companion*. New York: Prentice Hall/Parkside.

On father-daughter incest

Armstrong, Louise. (1987). *Kiss Daddy Goodnight: Ten Years Later*. New York: Pocket Books.

Brady, Katherine. (1979). *Father's Days: A True Story of Incest*. New York: Dell.

Camille, Pamela. (1988). *Step on a Crack (You Break your Father's Back)*. Chimney Rock, CO: Freedom Lights Press.

McNaron, Toni and Yarrow Morgan. (1982). *Voices in the Night: Women Speaking about Incest*. Pittsburgh: Cleis Press.

Poston, Carol and Karen Lison. (1989). *Reclaiming Our Lives: Hope for Adult Survivors of Incest*. New York: Bantam.

Ratner, Ellen. (1990). *The Other Side of the Family: A Book for Recovery from Abuse, Incest, and Neglect*. Deerfield Beach, FL: Health Communications.

Sessions, Shelly and Peter Meyer. (1990). *Dark Obsession: A True Story of Incest and Justice*. New York: Putnam.

On mother-daughter Incest

Evert, Kathy and Inie Bijkerk. (1988). *When You're Ready: A Woman's Healing from Childhood Physical and Sexual Abuse by Her Mother.* Walnut Creek, CA: Launch Press.

McNaron, Toni and Yarrow Morgan. (1982). *Voices in the Night: Women Speaking about Incest.* Pittsburgh: Cleis Press.

On sibling incest

Cole, Autumn and Becca Brin Manlove. (1991). *Brother-Sister Sexual Abuse: It Happens and It Hurts. A Book for Sister Survivors.* Ely, MN: Beccautumn Books. For a copy, send $7.95 to: c/o Sexual Assault Program of Northern St. Louis County, 505 12th Avenue West, Virginia, MN 55792.

On multi-generational incest: abuse by grandparents

Randall, Margaret. (1987). *This Is About Incest.* Ithaca: Firebrand Books.

Books for beginners: those just starting the healing process

Barnes, Patty Derosier. (1991). *The Woman Inside: From Incest Victim to Survivor.* Racine, WI: Mother Courage Press.

Daugherty, Lynn B. (1984). *Why me? Help for Victims of Child Sexual Abuse (Even if They are Adults Now).* Racine, WI: Mother Courage Press.

Davis, Nancy. *Therapeutic Stories to Heal Abused Children.* Self-published. For a copy, write to Nancy at: 6178 Oxon Hill Road, Suite 306, Oxon Hill, MD 20745

Gil, Eliana. (1983). *Outgrowing the Pain: A Book for and about Adults Abused as Children.* San Francisco: Launch Press.

Grubman-Black, Stephen. (1990). *Broken Boys/Mending Men: Recovery from Child Sexual Abuse.* Blue Ridge Summit, PA: Tab Books.

Lew, Mike. (1990). *Victims No Longer: Men Recovering from Incest and Other Sexual Child Abuse.* New York: Harper & Row.

Books for the advanced: graphic portrayals of survival

Danica, Elly. (1988). *Don't. A Woman's Word.* Pittsburgh: Cleis Press.

White, Louise. (1988). *The Obsidian Mirror: An Adult Healing from Incest.* Seattle: Seal Press.

Books written especially for survivors of rape

Adams, Caren and Jennifer Fay. (1989). *Free of the Shadows: Recovering from Sexual Violence.* Oakland, CA: New Harbinger Publ.

Johnson, Kathryn M. (?). *If you are raped.*

Ledray, Linda. (1986). *Recovering from Rape.* New York: Henry Holt & Co.

Los Angeles Commission on Assaults Against Women. (1991). *Surviving Sexual Assault.* Chicago: Congdon & Weed.

Warshaw, Robin. (1988). *I Never Called it Rape... The Ms. Report on recognizing, fighting, and surviving date and acquaintance rape.* New York: Harper & Row.

Books written for survivors of ritual abuse

Hassan, Steven. (1988). *Combating Mind Control.* Colchester, VT: Inner Traditions.

Kahaner, Larry. (1988). *Cults that Kill.* New York: Warner Books. Note: Graphic depictions of ritual abuse are included.

LA County Commission for Women. (1989). *Ritual Abuse: Definitions, Glossary, and the Use of Mind Control.* For a copy, send $5.00 to: 383 Hall of Administration, 500 W. Temple St. Los Angeles, CA 90012.

Smith, Michelle and Lawrence Pazder. (1987). *Michelle Remembers.* New York: Pocket Books.

Spencer, Judith. (1989). *Suffer the Child.* New York: Pocket Books.

Stardancer, L.J. *Turtleboy and Jet the Wonderpup! A Therapeutic Comic for Ritual Abuse Survivors.* For a copy, send $7.00 to: P.O. Box 1284, Lakesport, CA 95453.

Recovery from abuse with 12-Step approaches

McClure, Mary Beth. (1990). *Reclaiming the Heart: A Handbook for Help and Hope for Survivors of Incest.* New York: Warner Books.

Sanders, Timothy. (1991). *Healing the Wounded Child: A 12-Step Recovery Program for Adult Male Survivors of Child Sexual Abuse.* Freedom, CA: Crossing Press.

Thomas, T. (1990). *Men Surviving Incest: A Survivor Shares the Recovery Process.* Walnut Creek, CA: Launch Press.

Research on sexual abuse

For some, workbooks and guidelines are not enough: they want the hardcore research and statistics on child and adolescent sexual abuse. The advanced layperson and clinician may find additional information in the books listed below:

Bolton, Frank, Larry Morris and Ann McEachron. (1989). *Males at Risk: The Other Side of Child Sexual Abuse.* Newbury Park, CA: Sage Publications.

Burson, Malcolm. (1990). *Discerning the Call to Social Ministry. An Alban Institute Case Study in Congregational Outreach.* Washington, D.C.: The Alban Institute.

Butler, Sandra. (1985). *Conspiracy of Silence: The Trauma of Incest.* San Francisco: Volcano Press.

Courtois, Christine A. (1988). *Healing the Incest Wound: Adult Survivors in Therapy.* New York: W.W. Norton & Co.

Crewsdon, John. (1989). *By Silence Betrayed: Sexual Abuse of Children in America.* New York: Little, Brown & Co.

Finklehor, David.(1979). *Sexually Victimized Children.* New York: Free Press. (1984). *Child Sexual Abuse: New Theory and Research.* New York: Free Press. (1985). *License to Rape: Sexual Abuse of Wives.* New York: Free Press.

Finklehor, David, ed. (1986). *A Sourcebook on Child Sexual Abuse.* Beverly Hills, CA: Sage Publications.

Gelinas, D.J. (1983). *The persisting negative effects of incest.* Psychiatry, 46, pps. 312-332.

Hechsler, David. (1989). *The Battle and the Backlash: The Child Sexual Abuse War.* Lexington, MA: Lexington Books.

Herman, Judith. (1981). *Father-Daughter Incest.* Cambridge: Harvard University Press.

Hunter, Mic. (1990). *Sexually Abused Boys.* Lexington, MA: Lexington Books. The Sexually Abused Male, volumes 1 & 2. Lexington, MA: Lexington Books.

Maltz, Wendy and Beverly Holman. (1987). *Incest and Sexuality.* Lexington, MA: Lexington Books, D.C. Heath & Co.

Patton, Michael Q., ed. (1991). *Family Sexual Abuse: Frontline Research and Evaluation.* Newbury Park, CA: Sage.

Rush, Florence. (1980). *The Best Kept Secret: Sexual Abuse of Children.* Englewood Cliffs, NJ: Prentice-Hall.

Russell, Diana. (1986). *The Secret Trauma: Incest in the Lives of Girls and Women.* New York: Basic Books.

Books written on sexual abuse for and about the clergy

Fortune, Marie. (1983). *Sexual Violence: The Unmentionable Sin: An Ethical and Pastoral Perspective.* New York: Pilgrim Press.

Pellauer, Mary, Barbara Chester, and Jane Boyajian. (1986). *Sexual Assault and Abuse: A Handbook for Clergy and Religious Professionals.* San Francisco: Harper & Row.

Rossetti, Stephen. (1990). *Slayer of the Soul: Child Sexual Abuse and the Catholic Church.* Mystic, CT: Twenty-third Publications.

Newsletters & Journals

B.E.A.M. (Being Energetic About Multiplicity). An expressive forum for survivors with Multiple Personality Disorder. Write to: P.O. Box 1776, Cahokia, IL 62206-1776

Beyond Survival. A magazine and network for survivors of all kinds of abuse. Write: 1278 Gleneyre St., #3, Laguna Beach, CA 92651 or call: (714) 563-6330

Dissociation. The professional journal of ISSMP&D. c/o Ridgeview Institute, 3995 So. Cobb D. Smyrna, GA 30080-6397. (404) 333-0638

First Class Male. A quarterly newsletter for male survivors of sexual abuse and their allies in healing. Write: 50 N. Arlington Avenue, Indianapolis, IN 46219

For Crying Out Loud: The Survivor's Newsletter Collective. A quarterly newsletter for and by female sexual abuse survivors. For more information, write: c/o Women's Center, 46 Pleasant St., Cambridge, MA 02139

Healing Paths. A bimonthly newsletter/journal for survivors. For more information, write to: P.O. Box 599, Coos Bay, OR 97420-0114

Incest Survivors Information Exchange. A newsletter/open forum for and by survivors of incest. For more information, write to: P.O. Box 3399, New Haven, CT 06515

Just Us! A newsletter which provides information to survivors with MPD and histories of ritual abuse. Write to: P.O. Box 1121, Parker, CO 80134 or call: (303) 643-8698

Many Voices. A national bimonthly publication for survivors with MPD or other dissociative disorders. For info: P.O. Box 2639, Cincinnati, OH 45201-2639

Moving Forward. A bimonthly newsletter for survivors and their partners and allies. Write: P.O. Box 4426, Arlington, VA 22204

MPD Reaching Out. A Newsletter about Multiple Personality Disorder. A newsletter by and for MPDs currently in treatment. For more information, write: c/o Public Relations Department Royal Ottawa Hospital, 1145 Carling Avenue, Ottawa, CAN K1Z7K4

Multiple Care Unit. Bimonthly newsletter for MPD. Write: P.O. Box 82, NDG, Montreal, Quebec H4A 3P4, CANADA

Serenity Quest. A Newsletter to Promote Growth and Healing. A newsletter for those in 12-step programs, including recovering survivors. Write: P.O. Box 2332, West Covina, CA 91723

S.H.A.R.E. (Support Help and Resources Exchange)/ The MAZE. SHARE is a bimonthly newsletter for partners and allies of those with MPD. The MAZE is a bimonthly newsletter for those with MPD or other Dissociative disorders. Write to: P.O. Box 88722, Tukwila, WA 98138

S.O.A.R. (Survivors of Abusive Rituals). A newsletter for survivors of ritual abuse. For more info, write: P.O. Box 1776, Cahokia, IL 62206

S.O.F.I.E. (Survivors of Female Incest Emerge). A bimonthly newsletter for survivors who were abused by significant women in their lives. Write to: P.O. Box 2794, Renton, WA 98056-2794

Stand Fast. A newsletter for partners and allies of survivors. Write to: P.O. Box 9107, Warwick, RI 02889

SURVIVOR. A Creative Journal Created by Men and Women Survivors of Sexual Assault. A sophisticated quarterly magazine written for and by survivors. For more information, write to: Redbaux Communications, 3636 Taliluna, Suite 125, Knoxville, TN 37919

SURVIVORSHIP. A literary forum for survivors of ritual abuse or torture. Write to: 3181 Mission Street, #139, San Francisco, CA 94110

The Adult Survivor. A bimonthly newsletter written for and by survivors of child abuse. For info: 1318 Ridgecrest Circle, Denton, TX 76205-5424

The Chorus. The newsletter available to members of VOICES in Action (see list of "resource groups" which follows). Write to: P.O. Box 148309, Chicago, IL 60614 or call: (312) 327-1500

The Cutting Edge. A newsletter for survivors who self-injure. For info.: P.O. Box 20819, Cleveland, OH 44120-7819

The Healing Woman. Monthly publication for female survivors. Write to: P.O. Box 3038, Moss Beach, CA 94038 or call: (415) 728-0339

The Survivor Network Newsletter. A quarterly newsletter written for and by survivors. For more information, write to: P.L.E.A., P.O. Box 6545, Santa Fe, NM 87502-6545

Trauma and Recovery Newsletter. A newsletter for professionals providing treatment of trauma-related conditions. Write to: c/o Akron General Medical Center Department of Psychiatry and Behavioral Sciences 400 Wabash Avenue, Suite 5400 Akron, Ohio 44307 or call: (216) 384-6525

Traumatic Stress Points. A professional publication featuring information provided by the Society for Traumatic Stress Studies. Write to: 435 N. Michigan Ave., Suite 1717, Chicago, IL 60611

Treating Abuse Today. A newsletter for professionals treating survivors. Write to: 2722 Eastlake Avenue East, Suite 300, Seattle, WA 98102

Women's Recovery Network Newsletter. This bi-monthly newsletter is for female survivors. For more information, write to: P.O. Box 141554, Columbus, OH 43214

Audiocassettes

Audio Archives of Canada. Audio tapes of conferences addressing MPD and Dissociation. For more information, write: 100 West Beaver Creek, Unit 18 Richmond Hill, Ontario, L4B 1H4 CANADA or call: (416) 889-6555

Audio Transcripts, Ltd. Audio tapes of conferences and meetings addressing MPD and Dissociation. Write: 335 South Patrick St., Alexandria, VA 22314 or call: (800) 338-2111

Bass, Ellen and Larua Davis. (1988). The Courage to Heal: A Guide for Women Survivors of Child Sexual Abuse. New York: Harper & Row.

Cole, Autumn and Becca Brin Manlove. (1991). Brother-Sister Sexual Abuse: It Happens and It Hurts. A Book for Sister Survivors. Ely, MN: Beccautumn Books. For a copy, send $9.95 to: c/o Sexual Assault Program of Northern St. Louis County, 505 12th Avenue West, Virgina, MN 55792.

Davis, Nancy. (?). Therapeutic Stories to Heal Abused Children. For a copy, write to Nancy at: 6178 Oxon Hill Rd., Suite 306, Oxon Hill, MD 20745

Fredrickson, Renée. (1992). Putting the Pieces Together: The Survivor Series:

> "Boundaries"
> "Victim-Think-What it is and How to Stop it"

"Sexual Issues for Survivors"
"Dealing with Your Family of Origin"
"Career Issues"
"Sexual Abusers"
"Dealing with Deniers"
"Grief and Loss"
"Parenting Issues"
"Surviving the Holidays"
"Shame and Codependency"
"The Lost Childhood"
"Depression and Anxiety"
"What Number Kid Are You?"
"From Here to Serenity"
"Building Healthy Relationships"
"Recovering from Sexual Abuse"
"Spiritual Issues in Recovery"
"Understanding Your Dreams"
"Improving Your Self-Esteem"
"Handling Emotions—Yours, Mine, and Ours"
"Don't Hurt Yourself"
"Sexuality in Our Lives"

Tapes run from 72 to 137 minutes in length, and cost $12.00 each. To order, write to: Fredrickson & Associates, 821 Raymond Ave., Suite 300, St. Paul, MN 55114, or call (800) 925-2180.

Underwood, Judy and Patricia Gaynor. The Isle of Pleasure: Tapes to Guide Women to Sexual Fulfillment. For a six-tape series, send $89.95 to Odyssey, 515 S. Sherwood St., Fort Collins, CO 80521. Note: Both lesbian and heterosexual versions are available.

Videocassettes

Braun, Bennett. (1988). "Ritual Child Abuse." For a copy, write to: Cavalcade Productions, 7360 Potter Valley Rd., Ukiah, CA 95482, or call (800) 345-5530.

Maltz, Wendy. (1988). "Partners in Healing: Couples Overcoming the Sexual Repercussions of Incest." For a copy, write to: Independent Video Services, 401 E. 10th Avenue Suite 160, Eugene, OR 97401

P.A.V.S.A. (The Program for Aid to Victims of Sexual Assault, Inc.). "The Bridge" (about sexual abuse in the Native American population) and "Boundaries: The Professional and Client Relationship." For a copy of "The Bridge," send $195. to P.A.V.S.A., 424 W. Superior St., Suite 202, Duluth, MN 55802 or call: (218) 726-4751. For a copy of "Boundaries," send $95. to P.A.V.S.A., 424 W. Superior St., Suite 202, Duluth, MN 55802 or call: (218) 726-4751

People Productions Video. "Speaking the Deadly Secret." For a copy, write to: 2115 Pearl St., Boulder, CO 80302, or call (303) 449-6086.

Resource and Referral Organizations

In addition to the books, newsletters, magazines and tapes which are available to you and your partner, there are many organizations which can assist you in your efforts to heal as a couple. You may find that you benefit from attending support groups in your area, or may wish to explore your issues together in more depth. Most people find it a little difficult to find "just the right therapist."

Some of the agencies listed below offer referral sources in your area. If you call the organization, they will try to locate a therapist or treatment center in your area, so that you don't have to pick a counselor at random. If the referral organizations are unable to find a counselor for you, ask a friend. If you know anyone who's been in therapy in your area, he/she may be a good source of information!

What if you're new in town and the referral sources aren't helpful enough? If this is the case, look through your Yellow pages for a listing of the hospitals in your area. Often, hospitals have units designed especially for the treatment of sexual abuse. You can telephone the various hospitals to find out if there are treatment facilities nearby. If there are, contact the director of the treatment program and ask for a referral for individual or group therapy.

If there are no treatment programs in your area, and the hospitals cannot make a useful referral, go back to the Yellow pages and find the listing of counselors, psychologists and social workers. Determine which clinicians are nearby, and then make some telephone calls. When trying to find a therapist, you may want to ask for a brief, no-fee interview, so that you can meet the therapist and ask a few questions, prior to beginning therapy.

Questions to ask prospective counselors:
- What are the credentials of the clinician?
- If your insurance covers psychotherapy, are there any limitations to the type of clinician that you need to see (i.e. some insurance policies will pay for you to see a Licensed Psychologist, but will not pay for you to see a Licensed Clinical Social Worker)?
- How much does the therapist charge, and how much of the charge will you be responsible for at each session?
- What is the specialty of the clinician?
- If the counselor does not specialize in the treatment of sexual abuse issues, has he/she had any experience with survivors and partners?
- Is the therapist aware of other resources in the community which may be useful to you?

- How comfortable are you with the therapist after interviewing him/her?

In order for your needs to be met, as individuals and as a couple, it is important that you both feel comfortable with the therapist you choose. While it takes most people a little while to adjust to therapy, you should have a fairly clear idea how you feel after three or four sessions. Remember, it generally gets a little worse before it gets better, and the work of healing from trauma (even as a co-survivor) is difficult.

Sometimes, outpatient psychotherapy is not sufficient to meet the needs of an individual. There are times when your counselor may suggest the use of medication, and will then refer you to a psychiatrist (a physician who specializes in the pharmaceutical treatment of people in emotional rather than physical distress). Sometimes, medication is sufficient to allow the individual to function better, at other times, it is not. In those cases, the individual (or both members of the couple) may need inpatient treatment.

Inpatient therapy is provided in psychiatric hospitals which specialize in the treatment of emotional distress or sexual abuse issues. If you need inpatient care, your therapist may refer you to a specific program. If your therapist can not locate an inpatient program for you, the hospitals in your area may be able to refer you to the nearest facility. Should you be unable to find a program that meets your needs, review the list below and contact one of the referral organizations. If you are interested in locating a treatment center for a perpetrator, The Safer Society Program may be of assistance.

Referral and Informational Organizations

Cult Awareness Network (CAN): 2421 W. Pratt Blvd., Suite 1173, Chicago, IL 60645; (312) 267-7777. A national organization whose mission is to expand awareness about the dangers of mind control.

DD-Anon Group One: P.O. Box 4078, Appleton, WI 54911 (414) 731-8546. A 12-step group for partners and allies of those with MPD or other Dissociative disorders. Can provide referrals for groups near you.

Electronic Conference for Adult Survivors of Childhood Abuse: c/o Button & Dietz, Inc., P.O. Box 19243, Austin, TX 78760. Available to survivors who are on-line with a PC and modem! This 24-hour bulletin-board is monitored by a therapist.

Healing Hearts c/o Bay Area Women Against Rape: 357 MacArthur Blvd., Oakland, CA 94612; (510) 465-3890. Information and referral source for survivors of ritual abuse. Conducts conferences annually.

Incest Recovery Association: 6200 North Central Expressway, Suite 209, Dallas, TX 75206; (214) 373-6607. These practitioners provide individual and group psychotherapy to sexual abuse survivors and their partners.

Incest Resources: 46 Pleasant Street, Cambridge, MA 02139; (617) 492-1818. This resource center provides clinical and legal referrals, information, and professional education.

Incest Survivors Anonymous (ISA): P.O. Box 5613, Long Beach, CA 90805-0613. A 12-step group for survivors of incest. Incest Survivor Information Exchange (ISIE) P.O. Box 3399, New Haven, CT 065151 (203) 389-5166.

Incest Survivors Resource Network International (ISRNI): P.O. Box 7375, Las Cruces, NM 88006-737. A Quaker-affiliated association whose mission is the prevention of incest.

International Society for the Study of Multiple Personality and Dissociation (ISSMP&D): 5700 Old Orchard Rd., First Floor, Skokie, IL 60077-1024; (708) 966-1024. An information and referral resource for survivors with MPD or other Dissociative disorders and professionals who treat MPD and Dissociative disorders.

Looking Up: P.O. Box K, Augusta, ME 04332; (207) 626-3402. This is a national support organization for incest survivors. Resources, referrals, seminars, outdoor adventures.

Monarch Resources: P.O. Box 1293, Torrance, CA 90505; (213) 373-1958. This is a clearinghouse for all kinds of information about sexual abuse resources. They produce a quarterly calendar of events for seminars, workshops, etc. on, for and about survivors.

Survivors of Incest Anonymous: P.O. Box 21817, Baltimore, MD 21222-6817. For listings of free 12-step support groups across the U.S. for incest survivors, send a self-addressed envelope and 2 stamps.

Survivors United Network: 3607 Martin Luther King Blvd., Denver, CO 80205; (800) 456-HOPE. A program of the Kempe Children's Foundation, providing support and resource programs for adult survivors.

The National Assault Prevention Center: (614) 291-2540. This organization works to prevent interpersonal violence through resource development, education, and professional training.

The National Center for Women's Policy Studies: (202) 872-1770. This organization studies women's issues and works to modify existing laws and develop alternative bills to best protect women's interests.

The National Child Abuse Help/IOF Foresters Hotline: (800) 422-4453. This is a 24-hour hotline which can be used to report child abuse and for crisis management.

The National Coalition Against Sexual Assault: (202) 483-7165. Survivor advocacy group provides referrals for survivors and families.

The National Self-Help Clearinghouse: The Graduate School, City University of New York, 33 West 42nd Street, Rm 1222, New York, NY 10036; (212) 840-1259. Listings for national self-help groups. The National Victim Center, Arlington, VA: (703) 351-5079

The Safer Society Program Shoreham Depot Road: RR1, Box 24-B, Orwell, VT 05760; (802) 897-7541. Resources and referrals available for both survivors and perpetrators.

The Sidran Foundation: 2328 W. Joppa Rd., Suite 15, Lutherville, MD 21093; (410) 825-8888. An informational public-interest organization whose mission is to advocate and educate regarding trauma-induced psychiatric problems.

The Survivors of Childhood Abuse Program (SCAP): P.O. Box 630, Hollywood, CA 90028; (213) 465-4016. An informational and referral source for survivors and their allies.

VOICES in Action, Inc. (Victims of Incest Can Emerge Survivors): P.O. Box 148309, Chicago, IL 60614; (312) 327-1500. A national support organization for survivors and their partners.

Webster, Linda, editor. (1989). Sexual Assault and Child Sexual Abuse: A National Directory of Victim/Survivor Services and Prevention Programs. Phoenix: Oryx Press.

Legal resources for survivors

Kelvin and Patti Barton: P.O. Box 7651, Everett, WA 98201. Note: After their own experiences with the judicial process and delayed discovery laws, this couple has become extremely well-versed in the procedures for filing suit against a perpetrator. They are an invaluable resource for those seeking to prosecute a perpetrator.

COVAC: 4530 Oceanfront, Virginia Beach, VA 23451; (804) 422-2692. Note: This firm specializes in survivors rights and legislation.

Greg Meyers: c/o Wise & Cole, 151 Meeting St., Suite 200, P.O. Drawer O, Charleston, SC 29402; (803) 577-7032. Note: This lawyer provides written guidelines for the survivor wishing to prosecute.

National Center for Prosecution of Child Abuse American Prosecutors Research Institute: 1033 N. Fairfax Street, Suite 200, Alexandria, VA 22314 Note: A monthly newsletter updates readers about cases and the legislature regarding child abuse.

NOW: Legal Defense & Education Fund Intake Department: 99 Hudson St., New York, NY 10013 Note: A clearinghouse for legal information and referrals.

Books written especially for parents of survivors

Byerly, Carolyn. (1985). *The Mother's Book: How to Survive the Incest of Your Child.* Dubuque, IA: Kendall-Hunt Publishing.

Golder, Christine. (1987). *If it Happens to Your Child It Happens to You! A Parent's Help-Source for Sexual Assault.* Saratoga, CA: R & E Publishers.

Hagan, Kathleen and Case, Joyce. (1988). *When Your Child Has Been Molested.* Lexington, MA: Lexington Books.

Sanford, Linda. (1980). *The Silent Children: A Parent's Guide to the Prevention of Child Sexual Abuse.* New York: McGraw-Hill.

Smith, Shauna. (1991). *Making Peace with Your Adult Children.* New York: Plenum.

Additional resources for partners and survivors

Books about Multiple Personality Disorder and Dissociation

Braun, Bennett G. Ed. (1986). *Treatment of Multiple Personality Disorder*. Washington, D.C.: American Psychiatric Press.

Kluft, Richard. (1985). *Childhood Antecedents of Multiple Personality Disorder*. Washington, D.C.: American Psychiatric Press.

Putnam, Frank. (1989). *Diagnosis and Treatment of Multiple Personality Disorder*. New York: Guilford Press.

Ross, Colin A. (1989). *Multiple Personality Disorder: Diagnosis, Clinical Features, and Treatment*. New York: John Wiley and Sons. (1990). *United We Stand: A Book for People with Multiple Personalities*. Walnut Creek,CA: Launch Press.

Books on relationships and intimacy

Covington, Stephanie and Liana Beckett. (1988). *Leaving the Enchanted Forest: The Path from Relationship Addiction to Intimacy*. New York: Harper & Row.

Goldhor-Lerner, Harriet. (1986). *The Dance of Anger*. New York: Harper & Row. (?) *The Dance of Intimacy*. New York: Harper & Row.

Hendrix, Harville. (1990). *Getting the Love You Want. A Guide for Couples*. New York: Harper & Row.

Schaef, Anne. (1989). *Escape from Intimacy*. New York: Harper & Row.

Woititz, Janet. (1985). *Struggle for Intimacy*. Deerfield Beach, FL: Health Communications.

Books and resources for developing your sexuality & identity

Blank, Joani. (1982). *The Playbook for Women about Sex*. Burlingame: Down There Press.

Eve's Garden: Suite 420, 119 West 57th St., New York, NY 10019. For a catalog of sex toys and aids, send $2.00.

Good Vibrations: 1210 Valencia St., San Francisco, CA 94110. For a catalog of sex toys and aids, send $2.00. For an additional catalog of their Sexuality Library, send another $1.00.

Hutchinson, Marcia Germaine. (1985). *Transforming Body Image*. Freedom, CA: Crossing Press.

Loulan, JoAnn (1984). *Lesbian Sex*. San Francisco: Spinsters/Aunt Lute.

Maltz, Wendy. (1991). *The Sexual Healing Journey*. New York: HarperCollins.

Underwood, Judy and Gaynor, Patricia. The Isle of Pleasure: Tapes to Guide Women to Sexual Fulfillment. For a six-tape series, send $89.95 to Odyssey, 515 S. Sherwood St., Fort Collins, CO 80521 Note: Both lesbian and heterosexual versions are available.

Wells, Carol. (1989). *Right Brain Sex: Using Creative Visualization to Enhance Sexual Pleasure*. New York: Prentice-Hall.

Affirmations and meditations
Brady, Maureen. (1991). *Daybreak: Meditations for Survivors of Child Sexual Abuse*. San Francisco: Hazelden/Harper.
Clarke, Jean Illsley and Carol Gesme. (1988). *Affirmation Ovals: 139 Ways to Give and Get Affirmations*. Plymouth, MN: Daisy Press.
W., Nancy. (1991). *On the Path: Affirmations for Adults Recovering from Child Sexual Abuse*. San Francisco: HarperCollins.

Fiction focusing on child sexual abuse
Angelou, Maya. (1980). *I Know Why the Caged Bird Sings*. New York: Bantam.
Barnes, Liz. (1985). *Hand me downs*. San Francisco: Spinsters/Aunt Lute.
Morris, Michelle. (1982). *If I Should Die Before I Wake*. New York: Dell.
Morrison, Toni. (1970). *The Bluest Eye*. New York: Pocket.
Murphy, Patricia. (1987). *Searching for Spring*. Tallahassee, FL: Naiad Press.
Swallow, Jean. (1986). *Leave a Light on for Me*. San Francisco: Spinsters/Aunt Lute.
Zahava, Irene. (1986). *Hear the Silence: Stories of Myth, Magic, and Renewal*. Freedom, CA: Crossing Press.

Publishers
The Alban Institute: 4125 Nebraska Avenue NW, Washington, D.C. 20016
Alyson Publications: 40 Plimpton St., Boston, MA 02118
The American Psychiatric Press: 1400 K Street NW, Suite 1101, Washington, D.C. 20005
Beccautumn Press: c/o Sexual Assault Program of Northern St. Louis County 505 12th Avenue West, Virginia, MN 55792
Cleis Press: P.O. Box 8933, Pittsburgh, PA 15221
Connexions Press: 10 Langley Rd., Suite 200, Newton Centre, MA 02159
Daisy Press: 16535 9th Ave., N. Plymouth, MN 55447
Nancy Davis (self-published), 6178 Oxon Hill Rd., Oxon Hill, MD 20745
Laura Donaforte (self-published): P.O. Box 914, Ukiah, CA 95482
The Falmer Press Taylor & Francis, Inc.: 242 Cherry St., Philadelphia, PA 19106
Firebrand Books: 141 The Commons, Ithaca, NY 14850
Freedom Lights Press: P.O. Box 87, Chimney Rock, CO 81127
Frog in the Well Press: P.O. Box 170052, San Francisco, CA 94117
Paul Hansen (self-published): 7548 Cresthill Drive, Longmont, CO 80501
Hay House: P.O. Box 2212, Santa Monica, CA 90406
Human Services Institute: P.O. Box 14610, Brandenton, FL 34280
Inner Traditions American International Distribution Corporation: 64 Depot Rd., Colchester, VT 05466

Learning Publications: P.O. Box 1338, Holmes Beach, FL 34218

Launch Press: P.O. Box 31493, Walnut Creek, CA 94598

Milkweed Editions: P.O. Box 3226, Minneapolis, MN 55403

Naiad Press: P.O. Box 10543, Tallahassee, FL 32302

Oryx Press: 2214 North Central at Encanto, Phoenix, AZ 85004-1483

Pilgrim Press: 475 Riverside Drive, Room 1140, New York, NY 10115

R & E Publishers: P.O. Box 2008, Saratoga, CA 95070

Red Rabbit Press: P.O. Box 6545, Santa Fe, NM 87502-6545

Robert D. Reed Publishers: 750 La Playa, Suite 647, San Francisco, CA 94121. Or call: (800) PR-GREEN.

Safer Society Press: The New York State Council of Churches Shoreham Depot Rd., RR1, Box 24-B, Orwell, VT 05760-9756

Seal Press: 3131 Western Avenue, #410, Seattle, WA 98121

Sidran Press: 11271 Russwood Circle, Dallas, TX 75229

Spinsters/Aunt Lute: P.O. Box 410687, San Francisco, CA 94141

Tab Books Human Services Institute, Inc.: P.O. Box 14610, Brandenton, FL 34280

Twenty-Third Publications: P.O. Box 180, Mystic, CT 06355.

Notes and References

1. Maltz and Holman (1987), p.38
2. Courtois (1988), p.6
3. Maltz and Holman (1987), p.12
4. Maltz and Holman (1987), p.13
5. Maltz and Holman (1987), p.11
6. Benward and Densen-Gerber, as cited in Courtois (1988), pps. 12-13
7. Courtois (1988), p. 89
8. Maltz and Holman (1987), p. 36
9. Maltz and Holman (1987), p. 8
10. Woititz (1985), pps. 19-20
11. Courtois (1988), pps. 332-333

Bibliography

American Psychiatric Association (1987). *Diagnostic and statistical manual for mental disorders*. Third edition, revised. Washington, D.C., American Psychiatric Association.

Bass, Ellen and Davis, Laura (1988). *The courage to heal*. New York: Harper & Row, Publishers.

Clark, Jane Cox. (1992). "Important basics about child sexual abuse," Hilltop Views, 1 (2).

Courtois, Christine. (1988). *Healing the incest wound: Adult survivors in therapy*. New York: W.W. Norton & Co., Inc.

Davis, Laura (1991). *Allies in healing*. New York: Harper Collins.

Fossum & Mason. (?). *Facing Shame: Families in Recovery*. Norton Publishers.

Gil, Eliana (1983). *Outgrowing the pain: A book for and about adults abused as children*. New York: Dell.

Grinspoon, Lester (Ed.). (1991). *Post-Traumatic Stress: Part II. Harvard Mental Health Letter*, 7(9): 1-4.

Lifton, R.J. (1987). *The Future of Immortality*. New York: Basic Books.

Maltz, Wendy and Beverly Holman. (1987). *Incest and sexuality*. Lexington, Mass.: Lexington Books, D.C. Heath and Co.

Middleton-Moz, Jane and Lorie Dwinell. (1986). *After the tears: Reclaiming the personal losses of childhood*. Pompano Beach, Florida: Health Communications, Inc.

Quin, Phil. (1992). "Child abuse from the inside out: People who survive and what is effective treatment?" Keynote address at the Whitfield County Mental Health Society, May 28, 1992.

Woititz, Janet G. (1983). *Adult Children of Alcoholics*. Deerfield Beach, Florida: Health Communications, Inc.

Woititz, Janet G. (1985). *Struggle for Intimacy*. Deerfield Beach, Florida: Health Communications, Inc.

About The Author

S. Yvette de Beixedon, Ph.D. has specialized in the treatment of sexual abuse survivors and their partners over the last decade. While she has attained advanced training in numerous clinical areas, she has chosen this field out of "love and need." She describes the process of healing from sexual trauma as "excruciating." She believes that clinicians who provide treatment for survivors and their loved ones must believe in the process 100%. Dr. de Beixedon has proven her commitment to the field by providing community outreach and education. She has presented her work at hundreds of speaking engagements and she has designed and implemented programs for the treatment of sexual abuse for several facilities. She has taught undergraduate and graduate level courses at several universities, she has written about sexual trauma and healing, and she has engaged in countless hours of clinical practice with survivors and their partners.

Working and training throughout the United States, she has enjoyed many diverse cultures and populations. Recently, she returned to Southern California after nearly three years in the rural South. As a survivor herself, Dr. de Beixedon is inherently aware of the needs experienced by survivors and their partners, and of the incredible energy required for healing. Her practice and writing reflect her deep empathy for those engaged in the healing journey. Her personal transformation enables her to present an optimistic and motivated approach to trauma recovery.

While her investment in the field remains strong, she perceives the need for balance and a healthy lifestyle. Dr. de Beixedon now maintains a smaller clinical practice so that she can spend time with her husband and four children. She combines the joys of marriage and motherhood with fitness, gourmet cooking, home renovation, and travel.

Book Order Form

Please include payment with all orders. Send the indicated book/s to:

Name:_____

Address:_____

City:_____ State:____ Zip:_____

Book Title	Unit Price	Qty.	Subtotal
Lovers & Survivors: A Partner's Guide To Living With & Loving A Sexual Abuse Survivor by S.Y. de Beixedon, Ph.D.	$14.95	____	_____
500 Tips For Coping With Chronic Illness by Pamela D. Jacobs, M.A.	9.95	____	_____
Chronic Fatigue Syndrome: How To Find Facts & Get Help by Pamela D. Jacobs	9.95	____	_____
Super Kids In 30 Minutes A Day by Karen U. Kwiatkowski, M.S., M.A.	9.95	____	_____
50 Things You Can Do About Guns by James M. Murray	7.95	____	_____
Get Out Of Your Thinking Box by Lindsay Collier	7.95	____	_____
Healing Our Schools by S. P. Mitchell	11.95	____	_____
The Funeral Book by C. W. Miller	7.95	____	_____
Live To Be 100+ by Richard G. Deeb	11.95	____	_____
Healing Is Remembering Who You Are by Marilyn Gordon (hypnotherapist)	11.95	____	_____

Enclose a copy of order form and payment for books. Send to address below. Shipping & handling: $2.50 for first book and $1.00 for each additional book. California residents, please add 8.5% sales tax. Discounts for large orders. Make checks payable to publisher: Robert D. Reed. Total enclosed: $_____.

Send orders to publisher, or contact for more information:

Robert D. Reed
750 La Playa, Suite 647 • San Francisco, CA 94121
Telephone: (800) PR-GREEN • Fax: (415) 997-3800